the MOST IMPORTANT LESSON

the

MOST IMPORTANT LESSON

What My Mother Taught Me
That Will Change Alzheimer's
and Dementia Care Forever

LAURA ANTHONY

NEW YORK

the MOST IMPORTANT LESSON

What My Mother Taught Me That Will Change Alzheimer's and Dementia Care Forever

Published in New York, New York, by Morgan James Publishing. Morgan James and The Entrepreneurial Publisher are trademarks of Morgan James, LLC.
www.MorganJamesPublishing.com

The Morgan James Speakers Group can bring authors to your live event. For more information or to book an event visit The Morgan James Speakers Group at
www.TheMorganJamesSpeakersGroup.com.

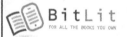

ISBN 978-1-61448-710-4 paperback
ISBN 978-1-61448-711-1 eBook
ISBN 978-1-61448-712-8 audio
ISBN 978-1-61448-909-2 hardcover
Library of Congress Control Number:
2013947439

Cover Design by:
Rachel Lopez
www.r2cdesign.com

Interior Design by:
Bonnie Bushman
bonnie@caboodlegraphics.com

In an effort to support local communities, raise awareness and funds, Morgan James Publishing donates a percentage of all book sales for the life of each book to Habitat for Humanity Peninsula and Greater Williamsburg.

Get involved today, visit
www.MorganJamesBuilds.com

Habitat
for Humanity®
Peninsula and
Greater Williamsburg
Building Partner

DEDICATION

For my beautiful, ever-present guardian angel and mother, Eileen, who taught me the true meaning of love, patience and kindness. I will forever miss you.

For caregivers and their families, who work so hard, love so deeply and sacrifice so much.

For God, who provided me with the strength and courage to relive so many memories and to weather the storm of emotion to help others on their journeys.

CONTENTS

"There are stars whose light only reaches the earth long after they have fallen apart. There are people whose remembrance gives light in this world, long after they have passed away. This light shines in our darkest nights on the road we must follow."

—**The Talmud**

THE END

> *"A man's mind stretched to a new idea*
> *never goes back to its original dimensions."*
> **—Oliver Wendell Holmes, Sr.** (1809-1894),
> American physician, poet, professor, lecturer, and author

Stretch…
Stretch…beyond current beliefs.
Stretch…to a higher level of understanding and wisdom.
Stretch…to a new beginning.

Congratulations! You've just taken the first step to a stretch in perception. You will never go back to your original dimension or beliefs. I've entitled this chapter "The End" because it will be the end of our current understanding of Alzheimer's and dementia patients' ability to communicate and pass on their wisdom.

My teacher, and yours, on this journey was a kindhearted and humble woman—an unlikely source for such a major shift in thinking. She never could have imagined that she would create a shift in perception or understanding about anything, let alone about Alzheimer's disease or dementia—a disease she didn't even know she had. But really, the stretch is even greater than that.

Maybe you are in the midst of your own journey with the disease. Perhaps you are trying to find meaning in your day-to-day activities while caring for someone with Alzheimer's or dementia. Perhaps you just happened upon this book and you are curious about the topic. In any event, I hope that through the course of this book you will reevaluate how we interact with Alzheimer's and dementia patients and realize the tremendous resource they are to us and to the world. As part of this incredible journey, I hope we all realize the significance of turning our memories into life lessons and using them to better our own life and our world.

After reading this book, you will be stretched to do the following:

1) Understand that the traditional wisdom regarding communicating and connecting with Alzheimer's and dementia patients may not be successful, satisfying, and life giving for many patients and their caregivers.

2) Implement a communication framework for seeking life lessons from a person with Alzheimer's disease and dementia.

3) Be able to confidently communicate with Alzheimer's and dementia patients to increase their sense of value and self-worth while providing a lasting legacy for yourself, your family, the patient's caregivers, and all of humanity.

Part I

FROM RAIN
TO RAINBOW

Chapter One

A BEAUTIFUL SOUL

*"What we have once enjoyed we can never lose.
All that we love deeply becomes a part of us."*
—Helen Keller (1880-1968), American author,
political activist, and lecturer

When I would lament about the aches and pains of growing older, she would say, *"Just wait; it gets better. Growing old ain't for sissies!"* That is so true, but how true it was, I was yet to learn.

She died on April 5, 2012—Holy Thursday. Part of me died that day, too. The coroner waived the autopsy. She was eighty-three. She had dementia and an array of other diagnoses. To me she was perfect.

She was my best friend. She was my soul mate and spirit guide. She was my mother.

I called her Ei—short for Eileen. My children called her Nana, and over the course of her last year, her name evolved to Nana Nu. I'm not sure how this came to be, but it seemed to stick, and she said she didn't mind when I asked her about it. In fact, I think she liked the whimsical sound of it.

She passed peacefully following her usual afternoon nap. It was sudden and unexpected. She was found on the floor in her apartment at the assisted living facility (ALF) by one of her loving caregivers. They tried CPR, but it was too late.

It was approximately 4:00 p.m. Dad and I were at my home. Dad was reading in the living room after spending several hours that morning with Nana Nu. I had just returned from a business trip that had taken me several hours away. I was deep in thought negotiating a business proposal when my cell phone rang.

I could see it was the ALF calling, and I was certain they were confirming my appointment the next day to pick out Mom's new room in the memory care unit opening in a few months. I thought about letting the call go to voicemail but decided to answer instead. *One less voicemail message I'll have to return*, I thought, as I was sure there were many others since I had been unreachable most of the day. Never did I anticipate what I would hear.

"Where are you, Laura?" the woman at the ALF asked. I said I was home, and she asked, "Are you alone?" *Why is she asking me these questions?* I wondered. I replied, "No. My father and daughter are both here, too. Why?" Her voice was shaking, and she told me that my mother was gone.

I fell to the floor in disbelief crying and saying it wasn't so. "She can't be gone! I loved her so much!" I screamed and pounded the floor with my fists as if the magnitude of my love should have protected her from death. My daughter Christina and my father came running from the family room. "What's wrong?" they asked. Still on the floor, rolled up in a ball, I pulled myself together enough to have Dad sit down in my office chair, and from a kneeling position and with a quivering

I screamed and pounded the floor with my fists as if the magnitude of my love should have protected her from death.

voice, I told him that his wife of nearly fifty-two years had died. This was the hardest thing I'd ever had to do; though, it was harder yet for him to comprehend what I had just told him.

He repeated my words over and over again as if believing that with each repetition, the reality of his wife's death would sink in deeper and make sense. My daughter Christina, who was only eleven years old at the time, stood in shock as she witnessed the entire scene. With tears rolling down her cheeks, she leaned against the wall for support—she couldn't move. She was speechless and scared.

I left in a voicemail message for my husband. "Honey, please come home. Nana's died! I need you." He was attending an after-school meeting with our son and had turned off his phone as requested. After calling my sister in Pennsylvania and relaying all I knew at the time, I asked her to call my brother and tell him. I just couldn't recount the story again, and I knew he would fall apart immediately, as I had done. I needed to be there for Dad. I wanted to go to the ALF and see Mom, and so did he. I thought that maybe then I'd wake up from this crazy nightmare.

I lived just ten minutes from the ALF, but the ride there seemed to last forever. Dad and I were in shock. My cell phone rang, and it was my husband Tom. "Please come help me!" I implored him. "I don't know how I'm going to get through this."

"I'll drop Ben at home and be right there," he replied. Always my rock, this time was no exception.

For the next several hours, I lay on the floor next to the most wonderful person in the world. I spoke to her and told her how wonderful she was and how much I loved her. Dad and I prayed. We cried. I rocked on my knees next to her side for so long that I had rug burns for over a month. I told her I wasn't sure how I was going to go on without her, but I knew that God would be waiting for her at heaven's gate.

I told her I was sorry she was all by herself when she died, and I prayed that she didn't suffer when she took her final breath. Oh, how I wish I had been there to reassure her and hold her hand. But the truth is that I needed her to hold my hand and reassure *me*. How was I ever going to get over this?

Now I realize that I never will.

How could my entire world turn upside down in less than twenty-four hours?

I had just seen her the night before and together with my son Benjamin; we had gone on a lovely walk around the pond on the ALF property pointing out the beautiful flowers and birds that were enjoying the picture-perfect evening as much as we were. She didn't want to go on the walk at first. She seemed a little tired that night after returning from dinner, but I convinced her it would be nice. I said that if she agreed, she could sit in the wheelchair and we would push her. We would make it fun, I assured her. And it was.

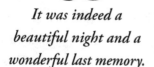

It was indeed a beautiful night and a wonderful last memory.

Most days she preferred to walk with her cane—the one her mother, my Nana, used as she grew older—and we reserved the wheelchair for times when we knew the walk would be long or when she was especially tired. That night met both criteria. "The fresh air will be nice and the sound of nature peaceful," we told her, and she agreed. It was indeed a beautiful night and a wonderful last memory.

Saying goodnight to her that evening will forever be etched into my soul. Not only did she seem calm and happy, but when I hugged and kissed her goodbye, she had the most beautiful look in her eyes. It was as if our two souls were touching, and for an instant, we were one. That's how it always was between us. When people saw us together, they would often comment that the connection we had was palpable. We had an extremely strong bond. We always did. We always will.

Ben and I headed out of her apartment door, and I looked back as she sat in her favorite green swivel chair. While waving goodbye, we recited our familiar parting words: "Now be good, and if you can't be good, be careful!" Together we laughed and blew kisses goodnight.

It was only twelve weeks earlier that we had moved her into the assisted living facility from her home two hours north that my parents had built in 1990 for their retirement. Now just ten minutes away, we were spending more quality time together again, and the joy and love in our relationship became stronger with each visit.

For the past five or six years, my visits with her had become more custodial in nature, and I missed the time we used to spend just talking about, well, everything really—life, people, good times, bad times, and everything else. Now living so close, I saw her nearly every day, sometimes twice a day, and I looked forward to getting back at least some part of our relationship from long ago—as much as possible, that is; I knew her dementia might hinder some of her recollections from the past. But that didn't bother me.

Even if I could just hold her hand every day, it would be enough for me. No longer would I have the four-hour round-trip drive nearly every weekend, the list of chores to complete before I left, and the constant worry about how she and my dad were doing. She would have dedicated caregivers to look after her and tend to her daily needs. *Yes, this is going to be good*, I thought. We'll both have more quality time—including time with my husband and my kids—for her and for me. This was my plan, though maybe it was not hers, and certainly, it was not God's plan.

As a child, and throughout my life, I looked at older adults who had lost their parents, and I wondered how they could cope. What would it feel like on birthdays, Christmas, and Easter, and every day, really, not to have your mother and father close by or just a phone call away? Could I fly solo if I had to? Was I strong enough for that? In my head, I knew that day would come, but in my heart, I didn't want to think about it. I knew that the day would be too painful, and I was right.

Looking back now, I realize the importance of those last three months with Mom here on earth. We laughed, we sang, and we talked about lots of things. These memories have been my savior during the grieving process. Not only have the memories brought me comfort; they have provided me the most valuable lessons I could have ever imagined.

Before moving Mom into the ALF, I, like many, fell into the trap of believing that she could not engage in conversation about the deep issues of life, and what she had learned over the course of her eighty-three years, because her short-term memory had failed her, and she only recalled stories from her childhood and early years. Somehow, I believe, with the grace of God, she revealed to me that wasn't true.

In some strange way, I wonder if perhaps by losing one's short-term memory, God allows the true essence of life to come to the surface. As far-reaching as it may seem, perhaps we have all become too preoccupied with the here and now—this day, this moment, this little snapshot in time. Maybe we are all losing the point entirely by focusing on the short-term and not seeing the bigger picture of life.

Perhaps the silver lining of Alzheimer's disease and dementia is that it forces us to focus on a much deeper level of humanity by connecting our experiences with life lessons. Ultimately, living our lives based on tried and true life lessons and passing those life lessons on to others is the point of life. Could it be? I'd

> *…the silver lining of Alzheimer's disease and dementia is that it forces us to focus on a much deeper level of humanity by connecting our experiences with life lessons.*

like to think so, and after my time with Nana Nu, I know so.

I would ask her what she'd had for breakfast, and she'd ponder for several seconds, but in the end she would say, *"Oh, it really doesn't matter. Whatever it was, I'm sure it was good."* The truth is, it really didn't matter. She was right. It was small talk and really had no bearing on the big picture we call life. But when I asked her to tell me the most important lessons she had learned during her life, she'd say, *"So many things, Laura. Where do I start? Let's talk."* She'd be as clear and sharp as a tack.

Feeling pride in our conversations, she was overjoyed that I asked. I was spellbound with what she had to say, and I never expected what I heard because it was always quite profound. She shared thoughts and ideas that changed my life and my beliefs about Alzheimer's disease and dementia care forever. My goal is to share this with you.

Here's Nana Nu's story. Perhaps it can help you on your journey. That's my hope. I know it would be Nana Nu's hope, too.

Someday, if God blesses me with grandchildren, I look forward to being called Nana Nu after a very amazing lady who was an angel on earth. Though I'll be Nana Nu number two, I won't mind at all!

In fact, I like the whimsical sound of it.

Chapter Two

CRISIS

*"The Chinese use two brush strokes to write
the word 'crisis'. One brush stroke stands for
danger; the other for opportunity."*
—John Fitzgerald Kennedy (1917-1963),
thirty-fifth president of the United States

I am not alone, and neither are you. If Alzheimer's disease or dementia hasn't affected someone you know or love, it will. There's a good chance it could even be you.

There is often confusion about the difference between dementia and Alzheimer's disease. The following will help you understand how they differ.

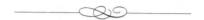

Dementia is a **general** term that describes a group of symptoms, such as loss of memory, judgment, language, complex motor skills, and other intellectual functions. Dementia is a condition severe enough to interfere with daily life. There are many conditions that can cause the symptoms of dementia.

Alzheimer's disease is a **progressive, degenerative disorder** that attacks the brain's nerve cells, or neurons, resulting in loss of memory, thinking, and language skills, and behavioral changes.

Alzheimer's disease is the most common cause of dementia (60 to 80 percent), or loss of intellectual function, among people aged sixty-five and older. There is no cure for either Alzheimer's disease or dementia.

If ever there was a word to describe the rise of Alzheimer's disease and dementia in the United States, the word *crisis* hits the nail on the head.

A crisis is defined by Merriam-Webster as:

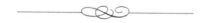

CRISIS

noun \'krī-s's\ plural cri·ses

1 a : the turning point for better or worse in an acute disease or fever b : a paroxysmal attack of pain, distress, or

disordered function   c : an emotionally significant event or radical change of status in a person's life <a midlife crisis>

2: the decisive moment (as in a literary plot)

3 a : an unstable or crucial time or state of affairs in which a decisive change is impending; *especially* : one with the distinct possibility of a highly undesirable outcome <a financial crisis>   b : a situation that has reached a critical phase <the environmental crisis>

The following statistics are found on the Alzheimer's Association website and are quoted with permission. To learn more, please visit www.alz.org:

- No one survives Alzheimer's disease. If you do not die from Alzheimer's disease, you die with it. One in every three seniors dies with Alzheimer's or another form of dementia.
- Today, an American develops Alzheimer's disease every *sixty-eight* seconds. In 2050, an American will develop the disease every *thirty-three* seconds.
- An estimated 5.2 million Americans of all ages have Alzheimer's disease in 2013. This includes an estimated 5 million people age sixty-five and older and approximately 200,000 individuals younger than age sixty-five who have younger-onset Alzheimer's.
- The number of Americans with Alzheimer's disease and other dementias will grow as the US population aged sixty-five and older continues to increase. By 2025, the number of people

aged sixty-five and older with Alzheimer's disease is estimated to reach 7.1 million—a 40 percent increase from the 5 million aged sixty-five and older currently affected. By 2050, the number of people aged sixty-five and older with Alzheimer's disease may nearly triple, from 5 million to a projected 13.8 million, barring the development of medical breakthroughs to prevent, slow, or stop the disease.

- Alzheimer's disease is the sixth leading cause of death in the United States overall and the fifth leading cause of death for those aged sixty-five and older. It is the only cause of death among the top ten in America without a way to prevent it, cure it, or even slow its progression. Deaths from Alzheimer's disease increased 68 percent between 2000 and 2010, while deaths from other major diseases decreased, including heart disease, the number one cause of death.

Impact on Caregivers

- In 2012, 15.4 million family and friends provided 17.5 billion hours of unpaid care to those with Alzheimer's and other dementias—care valued at $216.4 billion, which is more than eight times the total sales of McDonald's in 2011. Unpaid caregivers account for eighty percent of care provided in the community.
- Nearly 15 percent of caregivers are long-distance caregivers who live an hour or more away from their loved ones. Out-of-pocket expenses for long-distance caregivers are nearly twice as much as local caregivers.
- More than 60 percent of Alzheimer's and dementia caregivers rate the emotional stress of caregiving as high or very high; more than one-third report symptoms of depression. Due to the physical and emotional toll of caregiving, Alzheimer's and

dementia caregivers had $9.1 billion in their own healthcare costs in 2012.

Cost to the Nation

- In 2013, the direct costs to American society of caring for those with Alzheimer's will total an estimated $203 billion, including $142 billion in costs to Medicare and Medicaid. Total payments for healthcare, long-term care, and hospice for people with Alzheimer's and other dementias are projected to increase from $203 billion in 2013 to $1.2 trillion in 2050 (in current dollars). This dramatic rise includes a 500 percent increase in combined Medicare and Medicaid spending.

- Nearly 30 percent of people with Alzheimer's and other dementias are on *both* Medicare and Medicaid, compared to 11 percent of individuals without these conditions.

- The average per-person Medicare costs for those with Alzheimer's and other dementias are *three times higher* than for those without these conditions; the average per-person Medicaid spending for seniors with Alzheimer's and other dementias is *nineteen times higher* than the average per-person Medicaid spending for all other seniors.

These population trends are frightening, and they certainly scare most public health officials in the United States, including me. A dollar, a minute, a second, a person—many statistics try to sum up this crisis, but no matter what denominator is used, the bottom line is that these statistics represent a life—yours, your family member's, your friend's—and with each life that is affected, an untold number of lives connected with that person are affected. No one is or will be immune.

As the number of Alzheimer's and dementia patients goes up, the percentage of people in the lower age brackets who are and will be able to care for them is shrinking by a lot. This is even more alarming! These caregivers will need help. A new way of interacting with these patients (and gleaning their golden nuggets of wisdom) is necessary if we want to avoid a society of tired, burned-out caregivers and a healthcare system collapsing under the strain of helping these patients and families. We hope that there will be a scientific breakthrough in how to prevent and cure this disease, but until then we must prepare, and we must start now.

I know because I lived it. I was an Alzheimer's orphan. When I was caring for my mother, there were many times when I just could not be there for my own family. I missed many of my daughter's soccer games and my son's events, and my husband spent many nights alone at home. They were orphans, too! Even when I was at home with my family, I was unable to give 100 percent to them, although at the time I thought I was. The truth is I was just getting by most of the time. I was tired. I was worn out. I was trapped. But I had to keep going, and I did.

> *I was tired. I was worn out. I was trapped. But I had to keep going, and I did.*

Caring for me was not high on my list. I didn't exercise. I didn't prepare healthy meals. I rarely shopped. I did what I needed to do at that moment to get by. Occasionally, I looked in the mirror, and someone I didn't know looked back at me. I tried to keep up with my haircuts and sneak in a manicure or pedicure every now and then thinking that maybe on the outside everything looked okay. But the reality was a different story. I was gaining weight, not sleeping well, and worrying when the next crisis would occur. I don't believe anyone, including me, really knew the depth of what I felt during that time.

I'd speak to some friends about my struggles, and they would say, "I haven't seen you in forever. You need to do something about what's happening, Laura." My own husband and children would say the same thing. *What can I do? They don't understand*, I would wonder. *Why do they think it is so easy? They haven't had to deal with aging parents yet and all the feelings that surface during the process.*

Compared to most of my friends, my parents were much older—a result of waiting later in life to start a family. Most of my friends' parents were in their sixties or seventies. Mine were in their mid-eighties. I tried to explain that it was wasn't as easy as they thought, but I realized they were limited by their experience, and no matter what I said, they would never fully understand.

People I spoke with recounted stories of how one of their grandparents was declining and how their family was dealing with it. I listened attentively knowing full well that, in most cases, a grandparent's decline does not cut to the core of your soul as deeply as your mother's or father's does. You expect your grandparents to decline—you rationalize that it's the circle of life. They are older, and you have probably only known them as a middle-aged or older adults. Their daily caregiving needs were often handled by the generation before you.

In contrast, your parents are the ones who raised you from the beginning, and your memories of them are deep, profound, and lasting. They were the ones who wiped your tears and hung in there with you day in and day out through all the ups and downs of life. For most families in our culture and society, the care of the elderly falls first on their children, and most often on their daughter(s). This is not always the case, but it happens more often than not. With the transient nature of our society, adult children often reside in multiple states, and sometimes in multiple countries, which makes caregiving even more difficult.

Siblings and extended family members look to the caregiving children for updates, next steps, and answers. Unlike the generation before mine, extended families today rarely take on the caregiving role, and I wonder how this will change in the future considering that the birth rate has declined, and many couples have chosen not to have children—a topic for another time but nonetheless worrisome. In the end, I knew my friends and acquaintances meant well and thought they were sharing my burden, but caring for a parent with Alzheimer's disease is one of those things you cannot fully understand until you're in it or you have experienced it. Someday they may experience this with one of their parents, and I'll be there for them when that happens. Perhaps it will be different for them. I pray it will.

During the past several years of my mom's decline, my dad was in denial about it. He was always optimistic that some new medicine or vitamin would help her "snap out of the fog." My multiple attempts to move my parents to an assisted living facility or to bring in a senior care provider to help them were immediately shot down and never to be brought up again. My father always said, "Those places are for the old people," and as long as he could drive and care for Mom, he saw no need to even think about that as an option. Case closed.

Money wasn't the issue, as they had purchased long-term care insurance many years earlier and had even upgraded their policies with the annual cost-of-living adjustments. It really was just the thought of not having their freedom and not living in the beautiful house that they had built many years earlier that delayed the decision to seek a new living situation.

This perspective was not foreign to me; I had interacted with many seniors in assisted living facilities and skilled nursing homes, as well as seniors who were still at home. I worked in the home health arena for many years, and I understood how hard it is to grow older—at least from my naive side of the fence. I wanted to respect my parents' wishes and allow them to remain as independent as possible.

Having my parents at two different functional levels and not wanting to separate them made this an even more difficult decision. Mom needed more care, and Dad was still very independent and in good health. He was confident that she was fine at home, but I don't think he really understood the toll it was taking on me. Eventually her care became overwhelming, and the decision was made that something needed to be done. We muddled along with them still in their home, but we knew that eventually, perhaps sooner rather than later, that bridge needed to be crossed.

That day arrived. The straw that broke the camel's back came quite unexpectedly one week before Christmas in 2011. I had a business meeting just thirty minutes away from my parents' house. After the meeting, I drove over to their home for what was supposed to be a quick check-in visit to make sure everything was okay. My husband expected me home that evening for dinner—albeit a late dinner—and I looked forward to it.

It had been a crazy week. I was grateful for the opportunity to stop by their house because, perhaps—just perhaps—I could bypass the weekend visit so that my husband and I could attend the neighborhood holiday party on Saturday evening. Could it be that I had found time in an over-packed agenda? It was more valuable than gold! What I found, however, was extremely valuable, but not gold. That spontaneous visit changed the course of events in our lives forever.

When I arrived, it was late afternoon, and Mom was sitting in her green and white chair in the living room. The smell of urine and bowel incontinence hit me slap in the face as soon as I opened the front door. I went directly to my mother to hug and kiss her, and I noticed that the smell got worse the closer I approached. *Just put on your game face, Laura,* I thought. "Don't be upset in front of her," I whispered to myself. "She can't help it." I could see she was exhausted and exasperated about something. She was a mess. She needed a shower and a change of clothes. It was late afternoon—not a good time of day to deal with something like this. She suffered from Sundowner's Syndrome, which made things even more difficult.

Sundowner's Syndrome is a disorder that causes symptoms of confusion after sundown. It is often associated with Alzheimer's and dementia patients. The confusion often causes patients to become agitated, restless, and difficult to handle. Mom often suffered with these symptoms at this time of the day.

When I walked through her bedroom on my way to the bathroom, not only did I see that she'd had an accident, but the remnants were all over the rug, the floor, and the walls. Her bed sheets were pulled off her bed and were completely stained. I could tell that she had tried to clean it up, or rather hide it, but there was no mistaking what had occurred. I quickly changed out of my work clothes and went to work cleaning up the mess. Tears welled up in my eyes, not only from sadness that Mom was in this situation, but because once again, I was dealing with another crisis with Mom and Dad. My life was put on hold *again.*

I looked under the sink to find cleaning supplies but found undergarments and clothes rolled up in a ball and shoved to the back as though she had tried to hide them. *When were these put there?* I thought. *I was just here a few days ago!*

My father appeared in the doorway of the bathroom. He had just woken up. He was unaware of what had happened and felt terrible that he hadn't noticed it before I arrived. "It must have just happened," he said. What would have happened if I hadn't come by that day? Would Dad have slept through the night? How would Mom have dealt with a situation that was unthinkable to her? Many scenarios ran through my head. None of them were good.

After a very long business trip full of meetings, I had walked into a nightmare. Out of pure exhaustion and frustration, I declared that was it. Things had to change. My dad was eighty-three, and he had always been reluctant to change anything. He never would consider an assisted living facility for Mom. I put my foot down now.

I told Dad that I was making a decision immediately—that day. I was firm in my conviction. I told him I was sorry for having to do this, but because he refused to see the reality of the situation, I was taking things into my own hands. I could no longer live like this, putting my life on pause and picking up the pieces. My mother deserved better, and I was going to give it to her. In order to placate Dad, I told him it would only be for a couple of months until he resolved his own health issues. I told him it was in her best interest and his as well. In my heart, I hoped—or better yet, I knew—that it would be forever.

The next morning I called the assisted living facility close to my home. I had toured the building multiple times over the past several years and obtained several of their brochures to show Dad. We had even toured the facility a few months earlier, much to Dad's dismay, but because of his refusal to consider it, the decision had been put on the back burner—*again*.

I knew it was hard to grow old and give up your independence, but at some point, you need to put basic health and safety first. The entire situation and its impact on everyone had to be considered.

It was the time to act; I could no longer accept the current situation as the status quo. I felt badly that I had to override my father's wishes, but I shouldn't have. It felt strange. Throughout my whole life, he was the one who made the decisions, and now the tables were turned. Was I being disrespectful? Was I overstepping my bounds? No, I wasn't. This was a tremendous departure from the past; I was now the decision-maker and the safety net. It was scary and unsettling for me, but I trusted in the process and prayed for guidance.

My wonderful and reassuring contact person at the facility informed me that they were full and had no available rooms. My heart sank. *Now what?* I thought. She said they might have an apartment opening soon, but there were no guarantees. I knew she felt bad telling me this, as she was well aware of the uphill struggle I had been dealing with for some time. "We will be opening our memory care unit soon, and many rooms will be available then," she explained, but the fire was hot, and I had to act now. This is where I wanted my mom to live. It was a beautiful place with loving staff for both residents and their families. There weren't any other places close to my home, and I didn't have time to look elsewhere. My mind raced in many different directions as I tried to figure out my next steps.

An hour later, they called back and told me that their sister facility just two towns south from my home did have an apartment available, and as soon as an apartment became available in their building, we could relocate her there. The worst-case scenario was that we would have to move her into their new memory care building in a few months. I wasn't keen on all the potential moves, but I was very eager for an immediate solution and a proposed long-term plan.

"We'll take it!" I said. I hadn't seen it in person myself, but they alleviated my fears when they said the facility looked the same as their building, and it was managed in the same fashion. When I looked online, I couldn't tell the buildings apart. I called the administrator at the sister ALF and had a wonderful conversation that reassured me that Mom would be well cared for there. They tried to ascertain which apartment floor plan would be best for Mom. I didn't really care. I just wanted a new beginning. I knew she would be in good hands, and that's all that mattered to me.

All day I made phone calls. Some calls I even made in my car from my cell phone so as not to let me my mother overhear the conversation and cause her alarm. My father just watched me buzz around all day, but knew better than to try to talk me out of it. My siblings were supportive with the decision and agreed it was time for a change—if not overdue. To my mother, it was just another day. I don't think she even realized what was going on, and that's the way I wanted it—at the time. I decided that I would sit her down later and explain what would happen next once I had all my ducks in a row. Presenting a cohesive plan with confidence and resolve would be important to Mom. Otherwise, she might sense my trepidation and become fearful.

As soon as I was able to confirm her apartment in the ALF, I opened the locked boxes where she kept all their important papers and quickly found the envelope labeled *Important—Long-Term Care Insurance* in Mom's handwriting. Mom had sat me down years earlier and had shown me where all the important papers were kept. In fact, she had told me each time I visited her. I think it was etched in my mind. I was so thankful now that she had done that.

As she sat working on her word search puzzle oblivious to the happenings around her, this was exactly the moment she knew would come someday, and once again, she was spot on!

I called the issuing company and spoke immediately with the customer service representative who confirmed that both my parents had active policies that had been upgraded over the years when the cost of living indexes changed. That was Mom—always a diligent planner. Yes, my mother was covered for a fairly large percentage of the assisted living cost as long as she met the criteria. I was certain that would not be a problem, and it wasn't. The remaining costs were within reach for us, so we were incredibly lucky in this regard. Many, I know, aren't so lucky when the time comes, as the average assisted living facility can easily cost more than $5,000 a month.

I went into overdrive. I started packing my mother's things once I confirmed that I would be moving her into the apartment between Christmas and New Year's Day. I called a local furniture company and ordered a new bed and a couple of pieces of living room furniture to be delivered prior to her move-in date. I called my husband, and he was thrilled that finally there would be a change. Since we also had just moved into a new home, he dug through boxes to find pictures we could hang on her walls and lamps to put on the tables. My husband Tom is definitely a planner and was eager to help create a lovely, new apartment for her. He so loved Nanu Nu, too.

With the wheels of change moving quickly, I knew it was time to sit Mom down and tell her what was about to happen. I knew she wouldn't remember what I was about to tell her, but knew if I presented it with much enthusiasm and support, she would be excited too. I sat Mom and Dad down in the living room and told her that she would soon be living right near me, and we would be able to see each other almost every day. She was so happy about that. I told her about all the things we would be able to do together, like taking a ride to the beach to watch the waves, going out for lunch, having barbecues at my house, going to her grandkids' concerts, and just talking and spending more time together. She was thrilled! She said she was getting bored at home, and it would be a great change. Then she returned to her word search book and asked what was for lunch.

I packed my car full with as much stuff as I could fit in it. I also went to her primary care physician's office and had copies made of her medical chart. I informed them that she would now be living in an ALF two and a half hours away, and I asked if they would sign any needed documentation for coverage. "Absolutely," they said, and they commented that they were glad for her, for my dad, and for me. It was a big decision, and they recognized the courage it took to make it.

Next, I called the facility to see if they could recommend a local physician for her care. They did, and I called to set up a new patient visit. All this took place within a couple of days. What began as a quick check-in visit turned into a cascade of life-changing decisions. It was time. It was overdue. The next chapter was about to begin, and I was turning the page.

Many months later, I was second guessing the decision to move her to the ALF. I wondered if we had done the right thing. I guess it was that little voice inside that always wants approval and confirmation that we've done the right thing. I concluded, however, that Mom would have agreed wholeheartedly. Why else would she have purchased the long-term care policies in the first place? She never would have wanted to be a burden. She even wrote the word *Important* on the long-term care insurance company envelope, which reminded me of how high she ranked it in the priority list of life.

I left reluctantly and went home to put the finishing touches on Mom's apartment, fill out the required documentation, and to celebrate Christmas with my husband and children. There was really no Christmas for me that year, but I put my best game face on. Dad assured me they would be okay for a couple of days. I prayed they would. The plan was to pick Mom up in just a couple of days and bring her directly to her new apartment with as much excitement and anticipation as possible. I knew that she often took on whatever emotion she sensed from me, so I returned a few days later beaming with excitement about her new adventure, and sure enough, she was excited, too!

The ride to our new beginning was stressful for me, but not for her. I assured her that she was going on a wonderful new mini-vacation of sorts and that it would only be for a little while. Little did I know how profound that statement would prove to be. She was dressed in the new outfit I had purchased for her, and I had brushed her hair and even put a little bit of makeup on her. It had been years since we had gone to this extent with her grooming, and it felt good. Her easygoing personality was shining through, and I thank God for the strength he gave me that day as emotions were running high for everyone.

When we arrived, everyone was waiting for us. They welcomed us with open arms, and I nearly collapsed into them with relief and exhaustion. The hurdles we jumped to get to this day were many. She loved her new apartment, and so did I. I looked around it with a sigh of relief.

A few days later, we celebrated New Year's Eve in her new home. *How ironic*, I thought at the time. *It really is a new year!*

Chapter Three

TRADITIONAL WISDOM

"What you need to know about the past is that no matter what has happened, it has all worked together to bring you to this very moment. And this is the moment you can choose to make everything new—right now."
—Author Unknown

*W*hen you meet one Alzheimer's or dementia patient, you've met <u>one</u> Alzheimer's or dementia patient. This twist on a familiar saying always caught me off guard but I've heard this multiple times over the years, and I agree. No two patients are the same.

As human beings, we are all individuals; our underlying idiosyncrasies and personality traits remain a part of who we are throughout life, and perhaps they become exaggerated as we grow older. Likewise, Alzheimer's and dementia are very fluid diseases. Sometimes it appears that the patient has declined rapidly and is getting worse. This may be due to an underlying illness, but sometimes it is just the nature of Alzheimer's disease. Sometimes the patient may have a great day or several good days, and you think that they are actually getting better and never really had the disease in the first place. Many days, however, are just like the day before.

There are other factors to consider that can affect a person's disposition and behavior: sleep patterns, time of the day, living situation, and diet, to name a few. The person you knew in the morning may not be any reflection of the person seated across from you at the dinner table that evening. And the roller coaster ride between morning and night just repeats itself over and over. This is why caregiver burnout is so extreme with these patients.

In order to create some form of structure, many healthcare professionals have tried to create care guidelines based on the stage of the disease. This is the challenge—providing guidelines for treatment and interaction but allowing individual characteristics to dictate the best and most appropriate path to take. Each patient is truly unique and must be treated that way. Each day is unique as well.

Not everyone will experience the same symptoms or progress at the same rate. The following seven-stage framework is based on a system developed by Barry Reisberg, MD, clinical director of the New York University School of Medicine's Silberstein Aging and Dementia Research Center. This information is from the Alzheimer's Association website:[1]

---

1   The "Seven Stages of Alzheimer's Disease" is derived from the Global Deterioration Scale (GDS) from B. Reisberg, S. H. Ferris, M. J. de Leon, et al., "The Global Deterioration Scale for Assessment of Primary Degenerative Dementia, American Journal of Psychiatry 139 (1982): 1136-1139. Reproduced with permission.

STAGE	CHARACTERISTICS
Stage 1: No impairment (normal function)	The person does not experience any memory problems. An interview with a medical professional does not show any evidence of symptoms of dementia.
Stage 2: Very mild cognitive decline (may be normal age-related changes or earliest signs of Alzheimer's disease)	The person may feel as if he or she is having memory lapses—forgetting familiar words or the location of everyday objects. But no symptoms of dementia can be detected during a medical examination or by friends, family, or co-workers.
Stage 3: Mild cognitive decline (early-stage Alzheimer's can be diagnosed in some but not all individuals with these symptoms)	Friends, family, or co-workers begin to notice difficulties. During a detailed medical interview, doctors may be able to detect problems in memory or concentration. Common stage 3 difficulties include: • Noticeable problems remembering the right word or name • Difficulty remembering names when introduced to new people • Having noticeably greater difficulty performing tasks in social or work settings • Forgetting material that one has just read • Losing or misplacing a valuable object • Increasing trouble with planning or organizing

Stage 4: **Moderate cognitive** **decline** **(mild or early-stage** **Alzheimer's disease)**	At this point, a careful medical interview should be able to detect clear-cut symptoms in several areas: • Forgetfulness of recent events • Impaired ability to perform challenging mental arithmetic—for example, counting backward from one hundred by sevens • Greater difficulty performing complex tasks, such as planning dinner for guests, paying bills, or managing finances • Forgetfulness about one's own personal history • Becoming moody or withdrawn, especially in socially or mentally challenging situations
Stage 5: Moderately **severe cognitive decline** **(moderate or mid-stage** **Alzheimer's disease)**	Gaps in memory and thinking are noticeable, and individuals begin to need help with day-to-day activities. At this stage, those with Alzheimer's may: • Be unable to recall their own address or telephone number or the high school or college from which they graduated • Become confused about where they are or what day it is • Have trouble with less challenging mental arithmetic, such as counting backward from forty by subtracting fours or from twenty by twos • Need help choosing proper clothing for the season or the occasion • However, at this stage, individuals remember significant details about themselves and their family • Require no assistance with eating or using the toilet

Stage 6: Severe cognitive decline (moderately severe or mid-stage Alzheimer's disease)	Memory continues to worsen, personality changes may take place, and individuals need extensive help with daily activities. At this stage, individuals may:
	• Lose awareness of recent experiences as well as of their surroundings
	• Remember their own name but have difficulty with their personal history
	• Distinguish familiar and unfamiliar faces but have trouble remembering the name of a spouse or caregiver
	• Need help dressing properly and may, without supervision, make mistakes such as putting pajamas over daytime clothes or shoes on the wrong feet
	• Experience major changes in sleep patterns—sleeping during the day and becoming restless at night
	• Need help handling details of toileting (for example, flushing the toilet, wiping, or disposing of tissue properly)
	• Have increasingly frequent trouble controlling their bladder or bowels
	• Experience major personality and behavioral changes, including suspiciousness and delusions (such as believing that their caregiver is an impostor) or compulsive, repetitive behavior such as hand-wringing or tissue shredding
	• Tend to wander or become lost

Stage 7: Very severe cognitive decline (severe or late-stage Alzheimer's disease)	In the final stage of this disease, individuals lose the ability to respond to their environment, to carry on a conversation, and, eventually, to control their movements. They may still say words or phrases. At this stage, individuals need help with much of their daily personal care, including eating or using the toilet. They may also lose the ability to smile, to sit without support, and to hold their heads up. Reflexes become abnormal. Muscles grow rigid. Swallowing is impaired.

So what does traditional wisdom tell us regarding thought processes and communication with Alzheimer's and dementia patients? It varies based on the stage of the disease. However, as the disease progresses from mild to moderate or moderate to severe, most experts agree that you need to simplify the method of communicating with the patient but avoid reverting to baby talk or speaking in a childlike tone.

Below are some key bullet points outlined in the existing literature on how to interact with Alzheimer's and dementia patients. Many of the bullet points are very helpful. However, sometimes the advice in the literature is contradictory.

- Speak slowly and clearly. Keep things very simple and don't expect much from the patient. Give one-step directions. Pause often to allow the Alzheimer's patient to absorb what is being said. Use your natural tone. Do not shout, since this may be interpreted as being confrontational.
- Talk about familiar, easy-to-understand topics. If you stick with the patient's favorite topics or things he or she

remembers or relates to well—the weather, what's for lunch, the ball game, or upcoming holidays—it will be much better for the patient. Discussions that require abstract thinking or a great deal of concentration—politics and current events, for example—may prove too complicated.

- Expect to carry the conversation yourself. It's not that the person doesn't like to chat; he might have difficulty finding the right words.

- Give the patient chances to respond. Offer choices. Encourage the patient to participate in the conversation. Do not talk about the patient as if she is not there or treat her as if she cannot hear and speak.

- Don't ask too many open-ended questions, which may feel like you are testing his memory. This may make the person frustrated and angry and want to withdraw from the conversation.

- Take time to find out what he is trying to say. Suggest words when the patient is having a hard time verbalizing what he wants to say. Use visual aids when you can.

- Ask only one question at a time and make it a yes-or-no question or one that has limited multiple-choice answers: "Which do you like, the robins or the hummingbirds?"

- Think aloud for the person. Become a running monologue of life so that the patient doesn't feel compelled to speak. "I just filled the birdbath with water. I hope the squirrels don't drink it all!"

- Identify people and things by name; avoid pronouns.

- Stand in front of the patient when speaking to him or her. Have the patient's full attention before you begin to communicate. Don't start talking from behind or beside the patient. It helps to have eye contact when speaking to an Alzheimer's patient.

- Use the patient's name often when you are speaking to her. Start each or every other sentence with the patient's name. Always use your name as often as you can to remind the patient who you are. This may help make the Alzheimer's patient more relaxed and attentive.
- Allow the patient to talk, even if what she is saying is not rational. Pay attention to how he or she is trying to communicate. He may use certain phrases or gestures that may help you understand his meaning.

Other traditional communication tips for interacting with Alzheimer's and dementia patients include the following:

- Maintain eye contact. Visual communication is very important. Facial expressions and body language add vital information to the communication. For example, you are able to see a person's anger, frustration, excitement, or lack of comprehension by watching the expression on his or her face.
- Be attentive. Show that you are listening and trying to understand what is being said. Use a gentle and relaxed tone of voice, as well as friendly facial expressions.
- When talking, try to keep your hands away from your face. Also, avoid mumbling or talking with food in your mouth. If you smoke, don't talk with a cigarette between your lips.
- Speak naturally, speak distinctly, but don't shout. Speak at a normal rate—not too fast or too slow. Use pauses to give the person time to process what you're saying. Use short, simple, and familiar words.
- Be positive. Instead of saying, "Don't do that," say, "Let's try this."

- Rephrase rather than repeat. If the listener has difficulty understanding what you're saying, find a different way of saying it. If he or she didn't understand the words the first time, it is unlikely he or she will understand them a second time.
- Try to understand the words and gestures your loved one is using to communicate. Adapt to his or her way of communicating; don't force your loved one to try to understand your way of communicating.
- When speaking to an Alzheimer's patient, reduce background noise such as from the TV or radio. In addition to making it harder to hear, the TV or radio can compete with you for the listener's attention.
- Be patient. Encourage the person to express his or her thoughts, even if he or she is having difficulty. Be careful not to interrupt. Avoid criticizing, correcting, and arguing.

In summary, nowhere did I see it written that Alzheimer's disease and dementia patients possessed the ability to communicate, reason, or share their thoughts regarding life topics—not memory-based topics, but life lessons. Traditional wisdom lumps all patients into one category regarding this. I assert that not all patients are the same! There are many patients who are not only able to talk about life on a more philosophical level but who desire and yearn for the opportunity to share what they have learned with others.

It may take patience and knowing when to seize the right opportunity, but I believe we are doing a disservice to them and ourselves if we do not take the time to uncover the hidden life gems that reside within many of our Alzheimer's and dementia patients.

Chapter Four

DISCOVERY
OF A LIFETIME—
THE WISDOM EQUATION

*"The only real voyage of discovery consists not in
seeking new landscapes, but in having new eyes."*
—**Marcel Proust** (1871-1922), French novelist, essayist and critic

*I*t all started by happenstance and occurred months before
Mom's move to the ALF.
I arrived the night before after a long week full of coordinating
between my husband and me in regards to our children's lives and
our work schedules full of deadlines, meetings, conference calls, and
travel. As was commonplace on Friday nights, I transitioned from

my work persona back to my parental caregiver role on the two-hour drive from my home to my parents' house. I often wondered how many other people were doing the same thing. I knew I was not alone, but boy, did it feel like it at times! I needed this time to decompress from the hectic pace that had come to be my life over the last several years, and stepping into the slow pace of my parents' world was often a nice retreat, although it certainly came with its own set of stressors and challenges.

Driving alone in my car provided me my own private retreat center of sorts. I would often think about my husband and children. I am incredibly fortunate and blessed to have a husband who was understanding of my situation and was able and willing to take full control of the caregiving duties for our children and home when I was unable to be with my family. There were many times he had to pitch in for me when I was either out of town or heading north to cope with an unexpected or urgent trip to the local emergency room or doctor's office. Without his support and willingness to roll up his sleeves to get things done, I probably never would have made it through this especially difficult time. It had become perfectly clear that elderly caregiving, regardless of medical diagnoses, was a family affair, and many people's lives were affected by it.

I always stopped at the same gas station on my way to fill up the tank. I even came to know and expect the same workers at the fast food drive-through just off the highway on my route. They were like my weekend friends, and I would look forward to their familiar voices as they took my order. I knew in some way they remembered me too and expected me on Friday nights. They knew nothing about where I was going and why. They didn't need to. I didn't know anything about them either, but our paths always crossed on the same day at about the same time each week.

I remember a time when they were running a promotion where you received a free commemorative glass if you ordered a certain item from the menu. When I arrived, they had given out their last one. It really was no big deal to me at all, especially considering that I was privileged to dine at some very nice restaurants with my clients. The next weekend, to my surprise, they had one waiting for me because they felt so bad about not being able to give me one the weekend before. I really was touched. I still have that glass, and I will keep it always. It's funny how many lives we touch in so many ways without realizing it. How profound and ever present this thought would become to me!

During my journey to my parents' home, I would mentally list all the things left undone from the weekend before so that I could hit the ground running Saturday morning. The tables certainly had turned over the years.

I remember when it was Mom doing the driving. She would often drive down to my home when her grandchildren were young and spend days visiting and babysitting. Over time, the visits became less frequent and shorter in duration. I would meet Dad halfway to pick her up when she decided she no longer felt comfortable driving. Eventually the visits stopped altogether. I became her caregiver most weekends providing showers and her personal care. She would not let Dad help her, nor the female nurse's aide we hired for a brief period. She only wanted me, and in truth, I wanted to help her.

Over the years, I had become a super sleuth by being able to look around for clues in their house that helped me to figure out what had occurred during the past week. Like most, they were creatures of habit, so it wasn't hard to figure out when something was out of order. For example, I could tell how their week had gone by the condition of the bathroom, the piles of clothes on the floor, what was in the washer and dryer, and what food was in the fridge. Phone messages scribbled on the pad next to the phone and new entries on the all-important calendar recorded all the events in their lives, such as birthdays, doctor appointments, holidays, family visits, and so on.

My visits became very task driven—cleaning, laundry, shopping, and doctor appointments. I missed our long conversations about life, and the laughs Mom and I would share about days gone by and who had won the Bunko game the night before. She rarely left the house now. She was afraid that she didn't have the energy to walk any distance, and she worried that her incontinence would be an embarrassment.

She was much more comfortable sitting in the green and white high-back chair in the living room and staring out at the beautiful blue sky through the sliding glass doors. The days grew long, and she filled them with frequent naps and an occasional word search puzzle if she was up for it and if it held her attention. She must have had over thirty different puzzle books next to each chair in the house just waiting for her to pick up where she left off the last time she sat there.

This particular Friday, my parents' home was very much the way I remembered leaving it the weekend before except the odor in the air told me that there probably had been several accidents during the week, and Mom had probably refused to take a shower. By now, Mom absolutely dreaded the shower, as most dementia patients do because of the unsettling sensation it creates. Even if she reluctantly agreed to shower, she would only allow me to help her. The list of chores I needed to complete before heading home again started to build in my head. *Just get back to ground zero like last week*, I would tell myself. *Focus on food, medications, and a safe, clean environment. Everything else will have to take a back seat.*

Dad awoke early Saturday, as was his ritual, and had the coffee made and waiting for me when I entered the kitchen around eight o'clock. I sat with him at the kitchen table with my mug full of coffee and the powdered creamer. I had grown to dislike this creamer tremendously over the past several years, but I had come to expect it as a staple in their home no matter how often I longed for the real liquid stuff. Some things just weren't worth the effort any longer, and I had to pick my battles. I knew Dad looked forward to my weekend visits as they gave him the opportunity for conversation about politics or stories he had read in the paper. Our conversations were outside the usual, oft-repeated, and sometimes tense conversations he had with my mother when she was agitated.

On the table before me sat the little white bathroom cups turned upside down and stacked five or six inches high telling me that my mother's routine of four daily medication doses had been likely given as prescribed and administered by Dad over the past week. He was diligent about that.

His creative way of getting Mom to take her meds by placing them in the small white bathroom cups warmed my heart: He wrote little messages with a Sharpie marker or placed small stickers of butterflies or rainbows on each cup to entice Mom's cooperation with taking her pills.

The message "Take me; I'm yours!" was my favorite. His excitement one Saturday morning was palpable as he relayed the story from the past week about how he found these "wonderful stickers" at the local card store and thought he could put them on the cups since he was running out of messages to write. This was especially poignant for a man of eighty-three who was a product of the Great Depression and who never displayed raw emotion or spent money on something as frivolous as stickers.

Once the cup stack reached a height where it was nearly falling over, Dad placed the cups next to the medication pillboxes that he religiously filled each week after picking up any number of refills called in to the local pharmacy. Each day, Mom would marvel at the

> *It worked, and we always looked for things that worked.*

cups as if she was seeing them for the first time because in her mind, she was. It worked, and we always looked for things that worked.

I was always keen to get a bird's-eye view of the happenings inside their home. My daily morning phone calls to check in always gave me a sense of relief that at least at that moment on that day, everything was okay—that somehow, we weren't operating in crisis mode, and I wasn't trying to figure out how I was going to rearrange my life to deal with it.

My heart sank if my calls were not answered right away or if Mom answered after several rings but didn't know where Dad was or what day it was. The worst scenario was when I would see several missed calls from their phone or area code during the day when I was either in a work meeting or landing in an airport after being away from my phone for several hours. My messages would download all at once, and my mind would work overtime with worry. I would envision yet another ambulance visit to the hospital because someone had fallen or wasn't breathing well, or some horrible nightmare that I wasn't prepared to hear about or deal with had taken place involving the local police or the neighbors.

On this particular Saturday morning, after the usual set of questions and updates, our conversation turned to the new topic I had been thinking about all week (and longer). I wasn't sure how Dad was going to react, but I knew it was an important topic to bring up: their living wills, healthcare surrogate, and power of attorney. In the event that something happened to either of them, we needed to know what we were to do. My mother was a consummate planner, and I knew that she'd had these documents drawn up by a local attorney years ago. I also knew where I could locate them, but with

Mom's mental decline, I knew that the documents should be revised and updated.

Dad was surprisingly accommodating and agreed that we should revisit what was currently outlined and perhaps meet with the lawyer to make changes as needed. We both agreed that we should include Mom in this discussion even though she would not comprehend the discussion or the decisions we made. We needed to alleviate her paranoia that we were doing something behind her back.

We also knew she would have to give her consent to any changes we made to the documents. Dad and I finished breakfast and agreed to speak together with Mom in the living room later in the day after she'd had her daily dose of coffee cake that she loved so much. We knew she would be in good spirits then.

It was nearly noon when we sat down with Mom in the living room. I was too nervous to bring up the topic. I didn't know what to expect. I was afraid Mom would become agitated and angry, and that the conversation would become a frustrating and exhausting episode of repeating what we were discussing without her really grasping what we were trying to explain.

So we began, and to our surprise, Mom took it very well. She sat tall in her chair and listened. Her face and demeanor were focused and engaged. I explained that maybe we should modify their legal documents to reflect that if something happened to Dad, then one of my siblings or I would become the identified healthcare surrogate and/or have power of attorney over the estate and their affairs. Mom was concentrating hard and then summarized what we wanted to do:

"So in other words, you are saying that if something happens to me, and I am not able to convey my wishes, then Dad will make medical and financial decisions for me, but if something happens to him, then you, your brother, or sister will make the decisions." I was floored. Not only had she understood, but she was able to recite it back to us! I confirmed that she comprehended what we wanted to talk about it. Without hesitation, she said, "Yes—I think that is a very good idea."

Perhaps the coffee was extra strong that morning—or the coffee cake was extra sweet! Who was this woman before us? Could she possibly be the same person who didn't know the year, the name of the president of the United States, or how old she was, and who couldn't manage the activities of daily life without assistance?

She did not stop there. She went on to explain why she thought this was a good idea. *Whoa!* I thought to myself. *She said, "You and your sister know a lot about medicine and healthcare. I think you would be able to ask the right questions and make an informed decision, better than I would be able to do."* Wow. This couldn't have gone better. Dad and I looked at each other and couldn't believe it. She was alert, engaged, and her thought processes were clear and concise. It was agreed that I would make an appointment to visit the attorney in a couple of weeks, and the documents would be updated.

For several weeks after this encounter, I kept thinking about how she was so alert and able to process this complex topic and recite back to us an articulate response with such clarity of thought. In all other conversations and questions after this, she reverted to her usual habit of repeating stories from long ago in her childhood or early adulthood and forgetting anything that had happened recently. *What happened?* I thought. *Is her brain working differently? Perhaps Dad has been right all along. Maybe we are turning a corner in her condition.*

I, like many, bought into the traditional model of believing that if a person's short-term memory no longer exists, and only some events from her long-term memory can be recalled, then she cannot have any reasoning or cognitive functioning abilities.

Could memory and reasoning ability be separate and distinct? Do we develop our reasoning ability from our experiences, which are stored in a separate part of our brain from our short- and long-term memories? Thus, Alzheimer's and dementia patients may lose their short-term memory and perhaps some of their long-term memories but not their reasoning or internal wisdom. I find such things fascinating but have no training in this area. I was just trying to figure it all out. I definitely have a habit of overthinking most things, and this was one of those things. It is interesting for sure.

Everyday life brought me back to reality but not for long. It happened again!

Weeks later during another one of my weekend visits, I found the three of us sitting in the kitchen together at the table having breakfast. We all were staring out the window, and, as usual, my father and I were discussing some current event topic that was being broadcast on the morning show in the adjacent family room. Mom was engrossed in her word search books and eating her beloved coffee cake. Neither of us really thought she was paying much attention to our conversation when she looked up and seemed curious about the topic we were discussing.

Without really giving it any thought, I said to my mother, not expecting much of a reply, "Mom, what do you think is the most important thing you learned during your life?" I thought this would give her something to think about for a little while—enough time to get the small task at hand completed.

I'll never forget her answer. She sat up straight, closed her word search book, and pushed her breakfast plate to the side. "You know, Laura, I really believe that kindness is the most important thing that I've learned in all my life."

She went on to say, "You never really know what another person in this life has gone through. They may have grown up with tremendous hardships and adversity, and the kindness you show toward them could make all the difference in the world. Yes, kindness is the key."

She had blown me away again. My mouth fell to the floor. *Where is this coming from?* I thought. Not only was she able to answer the question in a very articulate way, but she was able to provide justification and clarification to her response. *That's my mother; she's still there*, I thought. *Her incredible soul and wisdom still exist!*

Later that day, when I had begun my drive home, I called my family to tell them all about my visit with Mom. I spoke with as much enthusiasm and excitement as a new mother would when reporting that her child has just stood up or taken her first steps.

Mom gave me the most wonderful piece of wisdom—more valuable than gold. But the wisdom was greater than just her response to my question, and I truly believe this from the bottom of my heart! She taught me not to accept at face value what I had read and witnessed firsthand about communicating with Alzheimer's and dementia patients.

> *Mom gave me the most wonderful piece of wisdom—more valuable than gold.*

I knew I was on to something, so over the next several days and weeks, I thought about all the other questions I wanted to ask her. I realized that I had to be very specific and *not* ask questions that were memory based in any way because I knew that she would struggle with them and employ one of her tactics to hide the fact that she could no longer remember. But I was thirsty and longing for the relationship that we used to have. We had often talked about life wisdom before she began to decline, and I was excited that perhaps in some small way I could have that back. What a concept!

A New Approach

I decided to work on a new approach to interacting with Mom, and this required a shift in me—not her. Her wisdom was still alive and reachable, but somehow in our society, we have convinced ourselves that Alzheimer's and dementia patients do not have deep, heartfelt wisdom or cognitive functioning because they can't remember what they had for breakfast. This has left a gaping void—emotional and spiritual—of loneliness and hopelessness for caregivers and patients. No one is gaining anything from this approach. In fact, we are spinning into a deeper problem: caregivers' depression and death rates are often higher than those of the patients they are caring for. The emotional, financial, and spiritual burden is profound and documented extensively in the literature.

Given below is a graphic representation of our traditional thinking:

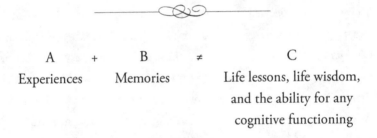

A	+	B	≠	C
Experiences		Memories		Life lessons, life wisdom, and the ability for any cognitive functioning

If there are no memories, then there is no wisdom or cognitive functioning.

The traditional belief is that if A and B are gone or impaired in anyway, then C is, too!

I wanted and needed to access the part of her soul or inner being where she already had converted her lifetime memories into life lessons and wisdom. I needed and wanted to get to C, but figured it was gone.

I loved to hear her stories (A and B), but the truth was that I was more interested in her life lessons and life wisdom. If I could access C, then I could harness that wisdom and come to appreciate and love her on an even greater level. My view of the world could be changed profoundly, and I would be moved to a much higher spiritual level in my own life where I could find greater peace for her, for me, and the place in life we currently found ourselves in.

I figured that when I moved to that higher level, than those around me would shift higher as well. Ultimately, we evolve our thinking, and life's purpose takes on a new dimension. Future generations benefit. This became my mission!

This lead to my discovery of what I call the Wisdom Equation.

The Wisdom Equation

Memories are special to us because they are linked to our emotions, and this link is what gives memories a special meaning. We cannot experience the memory of another person because we cannot experience the emotion the same way the person did at the time the memory was created. When a memory is relived, the emotion is too. Are we prisoners of our memories? Do they keep us from focusing on the lessons they offer us? Yes, I believe that sometimes they do.

Memories are important. Happy memories provide comfort and love. Sad memories help us to grow and learn. But memories are also a way to gain wisdom—also known as life lessons. Any number of experiences can create the core purpose of a memory or a group of memories. Our memories form life lessons if we are open and aware enough to heed them.

Over time, the life lesson can be repeated often and become a part of your life's purpose. Learning a lesson can be your life purpose. Memories are God's way of building a library of experiences to facilitate the learning of life lessons. Ultimately, this builds our life purpose.

Say, for example, that over the course of your lifetime, you have notoriously run late in every aspect of your life. When you were a child, you were always late for school, late turning in your homework, and late for soccer games and meeting friends. As a teenager, you were frequently late for your curfew. At first, you shrugged it off, but your trend continued into adulthood. You are always late on your bills, late arriving for work, or late on your project deadlines. The consequences were minor at first, but eventually you lost friendships, jobs, credibility, and financial security because of your inability to manage your time wisely. You are now perceived as disrespectful to others.

The lesson you learned was that not managing your time effectively ultimately affects your reputation and ability to earn a living. The lesson could form the basis of your life's purpose: For example, you become the inventor of an app that helps people plan their days effectively. You may have forgotten many of the early memories of being late as a child, but ultimately, the life lesson of being on time in all aspects of your life remains.

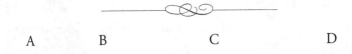

A	B	C	D
Experiences >	Memories >	Life lessons and life wisdom >	Life Purpose
		the ability for any	
		cognitive functioning	

Share the Wisdom

Just because A and B are gone or impaired does not mean that C is no longer there or able to be reached. If this is true, then D can be reached! We just need to figure out how it can be done.

Our culture is stuck on memories, and, boy, we are very good at that! We share our memories openly and freely, and with the advent of social media, we have become experts at documenting our experiences and memories in words and pictures for everyone to see. But we need to ask ourselves if we are taking our memories and experiences to the next level and learning from them.

As children, we learn that in order to walk, we must first place the weight of our body proportionally on our legs to stand up, but in order to move forward, we must shift that weight from leg to leg. The lesson is that we then know how to walk, but we don't necessarily need to remember all the times we have fallen down. The process of putting one foot in front of the other becomes engrained in our internal consciousness without us needing to consciously access the information.

There is no debate that caring for a patient with Alzheimer's disease or dementia is exhausting, but perhaps there is a silver lining we are not seeing. We must ask ourselves what we have learned from the experience of caring for someone with Alzheimer's disease.

My approach will not minimize the daily burden of tasks that need to be performed, but in time, it might create a golden nugget to cherish forever.

The most important lesson from all of this is to ask the life/soul/wisdom questions. Don't worry if the person does not respond right away. That's okay. It's a process. Pick another time to ask a different question. Ask questions that do not rely on memory, whether short- or long-term. Ask soul-searching questions about issues such as one's life purpose, relationships, health, money, and so on.

I am so incredibly happy that I asked my mother these types of questions. Whenever I encounter people or events that I do not understand or appreciate, it is such a blessing to reflect on my mother's wisdom. I would have loved to ask her many more questions, but our time together ran out. *I'll have more time to dig deeper into these questions,* I thought, *when we're all settled in.* Unfortunately, our time was short. I hope that your time with your parent isn't.

I am forever grateful for the time I had with her in the ALF. I believe the new environment gave us both a fresh, open, and safe environment to grow our relationship.

I often thought that perhaps her moments of lucidity were a fluke; perhaps I just happened to catch my mother on a particular day at a particular time that could never be replicated with other Alzheimer's or dementia patients. I thought I'd test my theory with others. On two very specific occasions, I had the opportunity to do this. Both patients were female and would be categorized as being in the moderate to severe category highlighted in chapter two. They were living in separate assisted living facilities in memory care units, so they did not know each other.

I asked both these women what they thought was the most important thing they had learned during their lives. To my complete and utter amazement, I received the same response from both! Each had me repeat the question and sat for several minutes before answering. But the answers did come—complete and articulate answers, in fact. The first one answered, "Kindness." I nearly fell off my chair. My mother had given that same answer! *This is so strange,* I thought, but coincidences are rarely arbitrary. The second patient told me, "The closeness of family." *Wow—that's amazing,* I thought. *I think there is something to this.* I had witnessed three moderately severe Alzheimer's/dementia patients being able to answer a very philosophical question.

I knew people would question my belief that Alzheimer's and dementia patients still possess the ability to comprehend and articulate responses to soul-searching questions. It went against all practical and traditional beliefs about the abilities of Alzheimer's and dementia patients to communicate. I figured that I would share what I know, and perhaps it would help others and possibly create a window of opportunity to think differently about this illness.

I've never been afraid to question things. In fact, I probably drive most people crazy with my propensity to overthink, overanalyze, or over-evaluate most things. I guess it's just part of who I am and how I tick. I have learned to keep it inside myself and accept that I will never understand it all. But this is one area where I believe that sharing what I've learned will pay off.

Below are some tips and tricks that I found helpful when speaking with my mother. I hope you find them useful. There is no right or wrong way to do this. Nothing below is earth shattering, but doing it with Alzheimer's and dementia patients is! As Nike says, just do it! Don't assume they won't respond, and don't let anyone tell you that you're wasting your time.

It will take time—possibly many months to complete. Keep it simple, but keep going. You may want to repeat it often with several different people.

> *"Simplicity is the ultimate sophistication."*
> **—Leonardo da Vinci**

How to engage an Alzheimer's or dementia patient with soul-searching questions:

1. Consider the timing. Typically, morning is best for most patients. Ensure patients' basic needs have been met: They've

been fed, they are rested and dressed, and they are sitting in a chair.

2. Create a non-distracting environment free from visual and auditory stimulation. I've found it helpful to make the lead-up to the question seem like everyday conversation. If there are others present, let them know ahead of time that you will be asking a specific life lesson question, and you would love their support in letting the patient answer in his or her words without being prompted. Encourage others not to interrupt.

3. Most Alzheimer's or dementia patients will take on whatever mood you display. If you seem upset, they will be upset, so remain calm, happy, and excited to hear what they have to say, and they'll be excited to tell you.

4. Have some questions written on index cards ahead of time if you believe this will help the patient. If handwritten, make sure the writing is legible. I always wanted the conversation to flow and seem like a natural part of our talk that day. I often had to repeat the question, but I would speak slowly and make sure Mom understood what I was asking.

5. Explain why you are asking the question, and tell the patient how important it is to you. Explain that there is no right or wrong answer. Explain that you want to learn from his experience because you value what he has to say. Reassure him that he is important to you.

6. Allow time for the patient to process the question. Avoid distractions and interruptions. It could take several minutes or longer. Don't hurry the process. Repeat the question if needed.

7. Let the patient respond without interrupting. The patient may say that she has to think about it, and that's perfectly

fine. Don't stare at the patient or raise her anxiety level by tapping your foot or pencil. Just be. Look out the window. Create a safe place.

8. If the patient seems disinterested or unable to focus on the question, quietly put the note card away (if you are using one), and perhaps try again at another time or on another day. Don't push it. The best conversations occur when they happen spontaneously.

9. If the patient does respond, you might want to record his or her response. Most smartphones have this feature. I also recommend using a notebook to write down the answer that the patient shares. Document the day, the time, and the place that the patient answered the question. Try to note the patient's demeanor. Take a picture to commemorate the moment and to thank the patient for blessing your life with his or her wisdom.

10. When you ask another question, be careful not to mention the previous time you asked a question. They probably won't remember it, and you don't want to get off on the wrong foot and put them on the defensive. Try having other people ask a question, too. This creates a wonderful family legacy, and everyone is part of the process.

I used several other communication tools with my mother that you might also find helpful:

1. **The Green Notebook:** Mom would always say that no one had come to visit her, or that she hadn't seen anyone in a long time. A certain green notebook became our way of documenting the day, time, and activity or discussion we had. It was a patient diary of sorts. There was no reason that it

was green other than that was the color I found at the office supply store, but we used it as a wonderful communication tool for Mom, the family, and her caregivers. Everyone in Mom's circle was educated about the green notebook, and we all referred to it when Mom was in one of her no-one-comes-to-visit-me moods.

When her home health aides, nurse, or physical therapist came to visit her, they left a little note in the book so that the next time I visited her, I knew they had been there. When I took Mom out for a ride to the beach, or to get an ice cream cone, I wrote about our outing in the book so that I could refer Mom to the entry later on and remind her of all the wonderful things we had done together.

The green notebook became a very important piece of Mom's legacy after she died. It reminded me of all the wonderful things we had done together, and one night, not long before she passed, without anyone knowing it, she opened the green notebook and read all the entries we had made over the past several months. She then made very special remarks about what a wonderful day it had been, or how much she had enjoyed her visit with someone. She made one very special entry, but I won't spoil the story and tell you here. You will understand it better in chapter nine when we explore the importance of humor in life.

2. **The Map:** Mom would always ask me where she was. She couldn't remember the name of the town or how she'd gotten there. She would also ask me where so-and-so lived and how far away she was from where she had grown up. So I went out and bought a map book of the United States. I opened the book to the page with Florida displayed and drew a star next to various places. I then drew a line outlining where

she was, where I lived, and where my siblings lived. Mom had always been good with directions. She enjoyed looking at the map and figuring out how to get from one place to the next.

I also opened the map book to New York State and highlighted the towns on Long Island where she grew up, where she went to school, where she lived with my father when they were first married, and where they lived when I was young. She enjoyed looking at the map and reading the familiar names of the towns. She would tell me stories about her upbringing and fun things she used to do. This was a very special communication tool for her because it grounded her in understanding where she was.

3. **The Whiteboard (dry erase board):** I purchased a whiteboard and dry erase markers of many different colors and placed them in Mom's apartment at the ALF. Not only did my children love to draw pictures on it for Nana Nu during our visits, but we would write messages on it, too, such as, "We had a great day today! We'll see you tomorrow after lunch. We'll take a ride to the beach. We love you! Laura, Tom, Ben, and Christina."

Not only did these messages provide a sense of comfort to her knowing that we would be together again soon, but they provided information to her caregivers as to when they could connect with us if they needed to.

There is no doubt in my mind that Mom would tell her caregivers that she hadn't seen anyone from her family in a very, very long time, and I know they did not believe her, but at least this way they knew when we would be back in case they needed to speak to us about her care. She read the messages on the whiteboard over and over again, and that told me she loved those messages. In that moment, at that special time, she knew she meant the world to us, and she did.

It might even be a great way for patients to communicate with us by drawing pictures or writing messages. Try it!

Everything in life is trial and error to some extent, so I'd also like to share something that did not work out well for us—at least not in the way it was intended:

The Phone Number List: Mom had a private phone in her apartment at the ALF. In order to help her speak with her family, I made a phone number list for her on poster paper using a large black marker. I listed everyone's name and phone number. When Mom was bored or feeling especially low, she would start dialing everyone on the phone list until she reached someone.

She would tell them to come get her right now because she wanted to go home. Often, this happened in the middle of the night. She would sound very panicked, which scared us all half to death! Then a series of calls would circulate among the family members until we made a call to the ALF and one of the caregivers would check in on her to reassure her that everything was okay.

I guess in retrospect it wasn't a terrible idea to have the phone list, but at times, it did raise people's blood pressure for sure. It wasn't long before I found the phone list during one of my visits, and I hid it under the placemat in her apartment. We all slept better after that, and she did too. Her caregivers learned to check on Mom more frequently during the night and reassure her that all was just fine.

In summary, the main point of this chapter is to encourage you to seek new ways to communicate with Alzheimer's and dementia patients and not let traditional wisdom block your creativity and desire to communicate with your loved one. I believe the deep wisdom and love they have is still there, and we just need to figure out how to access it.

In chapters four through nine, I provide key questions and activities for you to explore with the Alzheimer's and dementia patient in your life. These will provide amazing insights for you and create a legacy for your loved ones that won't be forgotten.

Part II

LIFE QUESTIONS, LIFE LESSONS

Chapter Five

LIFE

"*Life can only be understood backwards; but it must be lived forward.*"
—**Soren Kierkegaard**, (1813-1855), Danish philosopher,
theologian, poet, social critic, and religious author

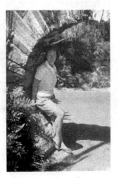

*F*rom the earliest recorded time in human history, an overarching question has perplexed countless cultures and generations all over the world: What is the meaning of life?

So let me answer that question now…only kidding!

This is a huge, daunting question for anyone to try to answer—even the most

Mom on her honeymoon in Bermuda. 1959.

intelligent, religious, soulful, and articulate person will struggle on many levels with this question. If you do venture into this conversation, you're likely to either be sitting for many hours delving into a very deep philosophical discussion, or you will be met with the shrugging of shoulders and a quick response of, "I have no clue," neither of which results in a deeper understanding of the topic or provides a sense of closure.

However, when you break this question down and personalize it, it's much more manageable and meaningful, and I believe it provides an amazing window to a person's soul:

What is the most important lesson you have learned in life?

In chapter three, I recounted the story of asking this question of my mother. I really don't remember exactly what propelled me to do this—maybe it was to create conversation, or maybe to give her something to think about. I'm not really sure, but I do know that never in a million years did I expect her to give me a coherent, articulate answer, which she did!

And what a wonderful answer it was: *Kindness.*

> *...who wouldn't want to know a little more about how to make life better, happier, and healthier?*

Life questions are my favorite types of questions to ask someone. They are broad enough for anyone to go in any direction they like and put their own personal spin on the subject; but they are specific enough that pearls of wisdom come freely, and general enough to resonate with most people. And, basically, who wouldn't want to know a little more about how to make life better, happier, and healthier? I think we're all looking for that.

Imagine how much our society, our children, and our world would learn and advance if we didn't have to relearn everything from scratch. In earlier societies, the wisdom of our elders was revered and actively sought. Have we lost our connection to passing wisdom from one generation to the next? Are we willing to allow a huge percentage of our population to slip away without asking potentially life-changing questions of them? I hope not. Let's start now!

Of course, there are certain lessons that each person must learn on his or her own through time and experience. But certainly, understanding how others respond to life questions places a great light on the subject and broadens our perspective immensely.

True to form, I couldn't help but look deeper into my mother's response to my life lesson question. She told me that being kind is the most important lesson in life. So what exactly is kindness? How is it different from just being nice?

Merriam-Webster provides the following definitions for the words *kindness* and *nice*:

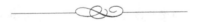

KINDNESS

kind·ness   noun \'kīn(d)-n's\

1: a kind deed : favor

2a: the quality or state of being kind

NICE

adjective \'nīs\

1 obsolete a : wanton, dissolute b : coy, reticent

2a : showing fastidious or finicky tastes : particular <too nice a palate to enjoy junk food> b : exacting in requirements or standards : punctilious <a nice code of honor>

3 possessing, marked by, or demanding great or excessive precision and delicacy <nice measurements>

4 obsolete : trivial

5a : pleasing, agreeable <a nice time> <a nice person> b : well-executed <nice shot> c : appropriate, fitting <not a nice word for a formal occasion>

6a : socially acceptable : well-bred <from a nice family> b : virtuous, respectable <was taught that nice girls don't do that>

7: polite, kind <that's nice of you to say>

The biggest difference I can see with these definitions is that kindness is a noun and nice is an adjective. Nice describes something, but it seems that kindness is more of an internal quality.

I really wanted to dive deeper into this, so I looked to religion and philosophy for more direction. Here's what I found:

- Kindness is the act or the state of being kind; it is marked by good and charitable behavior, a pleasant disposition, and concern for others. It is known as a virtue and recognized as a value in many cultures and religions.
- In religion, kindness is considered one of the seven virtues, specifically one of the seven contrary or heavenly virtues (direct opposites of the seven deadly sins) that is the direct opposite of envy.

- The Talmud claims that "deeds of kindness are equal in weight to all the commandments."
- The apostle Paul characterizes love as being "patient and kind" (1 Corinthians).
- Kindness is listed as one of the Christian Fruits of the Spirit by the apostle Paul in Galatians 5:22: "But the fruit of the Spirit is love, joy, peace, patience, kindness, goodness, faithfulness, gentleness, and self-control. Against such things there is no law."
- In Buddhism, one of the Ten Perfections (Paramitas) is Mettā, which is usually translated into English as "loving-kindness."
- Tenzin Gyatso, fourteenth Dalai Lama, wrote, "My religion is kindness," and he authored a book entitled *Kindness, Clarity, and Insight.*
- Confucius urges his followers to "recompense kindness with kindness."
- Basavanna's most-quoted saying in Kannada asks, "Where is religion without loving-kindness?"
- In Islam, there are many Surahs of Allah's kindness to his slaves. The Prophet Muhammad said, "Allah is kind, and He loves kindness."
- Analysts warn that "real kindness changes people in the doing of it, often in unpredictable ways. Real kindness is an exchange with essentially unpredictable consequences."
- It has been suggested that most of Shakespeare's opus could be considered a study of human kindness.
  (Source: Wikipedia)

What a wonderful gift my mother gave me! I can guarantee you that she never researched the roots of kindness and how it was reflected in various philosophical and religious ways. All she knew was to live it and see the results. Thank you so much, Mom! Your wisdom was amazing.

Asking life questions is a great way to find out more about a person's soul. I have listed several on the following page. Don't be afraid to seek out others or expand on a response you receive by simply saying, "Tell me more about that," or "What do you mean by what you said?" Of course, always consider a person's disposition, and don't try to overload a conversation.

Best of luck on your all-important journey!

Life Questions, Life Lessons:

LIFE

- What is the most important lesson you have learned in life?
- How would you define success?
- How would you define failure?
- What is happiness?
- How do you find happiness?
- What is your wish for humanity?
- How do you overcome difficulties in life?
- What is the best way to maintain balance in your life?
- What advice do you have for someone trying to find his or her path in life?
- What could the world use more of? Less of?
- What has always perplexed you about life?
- What is your ultimate message about life?

Chapter Six

RELATIONSHIPS

*"In your life, you meet people. Some you never think about again.
Some you wonder what happened to them. There are some that
you wonder if they ever think about you. And then there are some
you wish you never had to think about again. But you do."*
—Author Unknown

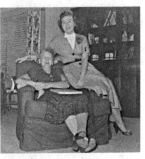

*My mother
and grandmother.
Circa 1950s.*

R elationships are important. They help us understand our world, our values, and ourselves, and they provide a framework for moving through life.

My mother's relationship with her mother was profound—just like my relationship was with her. One weekend night while I was visiting her, she fell asleep in her bedroom while I was still awake. I was in the guest bedroom watching television when suddenly, I heard her get out of bed, open all the doors to the closets, and pace frantically from one side of the house to the other.

I quickly ran out to see what was going on, and she said, "Where is she? I have to take her to the doctor. I have to find her now or else we'll be late! Where is she hiding?" I followed her around for a little while trying to soothe her. Finally, I sat her down at the kitchen table and asked who she was looking for, and she said, "Nana." I knew she meant her mother—my grandmother. I knew it from the first second I saw her pacing around the house.

I comforted her, got her a glass of water, and explained that she was just having a dream—a very real dream. I told her that Nana was already in heaven, and she was just fine. She looked at me and said, "But it was so real." She was staring at me with disbelief, and I could see that she was trying to reconcile the two worlds she found herself in.

I do believe she was reliving her past, but I also believe my grandmother's angel was visiting her that night. She so loved my grandmother, and I have heartfelt memories of my grandmother living with us on Long Island and the two of them having conversations at the dinner table long after everyone else had left—much like we had done for many years as well! I know that Nana was speaking to her. Perhaps this entire episode was for my benefit—to know that even after death, you never lose your connection with those whom you have a close heartfelt bond with during your earthly life.

On many other occasions during my weekend visits, I would hear my mother talking quite frequently, loudly, and articulately in her sleep. She would have full-blown conversations lasting twenty minutes or longer. Sometimes I could make out what she was saying, and other times I could not. I knew she was often speaking to her own mother, father, friends, and people she worked with over the years—all of whom had already passed. I often wondered if she was indeed speaking to those people in heaven, and they were preparing her to move over to that realm. Perhaps the talking was to reassure me that she would be greeted by her

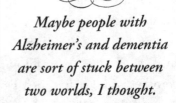

Maybe people with Alzheimer's and dementia are sort of stuck between two worlds, I thought.

many friends and family when she went to heaven, and I shouldn't worry when the time came for her to join them. *Maybe people with Alzheimer's and dementia are sort of stuck between the two worlds, I thought.*

On another occasion while I was visiting, I went in to check on Mom after dinner, and she was sitting at the end of the bed crying. I asked her what was wrong. She said she was so upset because she could not remember anything about Dad's funeral. She asked me when he died and where he was buried. I sat down next to her and put my arm around her. I hugged her with compassion and love (and a smile on my face) and told her, "The reason you can't remember, Mom, is because Dad hasn't died yet. He's in the other bedroom sleeping!" We both laughed. I made light of the situation, and I knew she felt better. Even Dad laughed when I told him the story the next day. Thank goodness, he still had his sense of humor, too! It really helped a great deal. She loved my father very much. They were married for nearly fifty-two years when she died.

Nana Nu was a socially outgoing individual. She always loved a party and having friends around. I have many memories of parties and gatherings with a full array of food, drinks, and lively conversations. She was so happy when she and my father moved from Long Island to Florida, which meant she could host her friends year-round on the screened lanai that overlooked the pool she loved.

Throughout the eighteen years she lived in Florida, she often had dear friends and relatives from up north visit for extended stays, and she missed them so much when they were gone. Books, cards, bowling, and crafts kept her busy, and of course, her dear friends Lu, Pat, Dot, and Dot (short for Lucille, Patricia and two friends named Dorothy) were her treasured Florida friends and co-conspirators on trips to Biloxi, Mississippi, or little weekend trips they would take from time to time. I often referred to them as the Golden Girls after the television show of the same name. I loved to hear about their escapades and what they were planning next. There was always something going on.

But over the years, her health and the health of the beloved Golden Girls declined, and the days grew long. Various friends passed away or moved up north to be with relatives when they could no longer manage on their own. The joy that was once so evident in her voice faded. Scheduling doctor appointments and jumping in my car with unplanned trips to the emergency room became more frequent and pressing. Her friends were my friends, and I too felt the sadness when one left the group.

Nonetheless, relationships are an important part of life. There is no denying that. We all learn a great deal from one another, so it seems fitting to understand how someone feels about the importance of relationships in his or her life. We could all benefit from pearls of wisdom in this category. The following page lists some great questions to explore this further.

Life Questions, Life Lessons:

RELATIONSHIPS

- What is the most important lesson you have learned about relationships?
- What makes a good marriage/partnership?
- What makes a happy family?
- What is the most important lesson to teach children?
- What surprises you most about people?
- How important are friends and family?
- How does someone be a good friend?
- What advice do you have for spouses, parents, and grandparents?
- Why do so many people struggle with relationships?
- What is the best way to deal with difficult relationships?
- What has always perplexed you about people?
- What is your overall message about relationships?

Chapter Seven

RELIGION AND FAITH

"The purpose of all major religious traditions is not to
construct big temples on the outside, but to create temples
of goodness and compassion inside, in our hearts."
—**Tenzin Gyatso** (1935–), 14th Dalai Lama

*I*t wasn't surprising that she died on Holy Thursday. She was a
woman of incredible faith in a quiet and gentle way. She was
Catholic, and being called home to heaven on the day we celebrated
Jesus's last supper with his disciples seemed appropriate and fitting. It
was as if Jesus was calling her home.

She was born to Swedish and Irish immigrants, and was raised
on Long Island with her three brothers. She attended Catholic school
from the primary grades to high school graduation. She married

my father in 1959, raised three children, and remained active in the church throughout her life, both on Long Island where I was raised and in Florida where she retired in 1990.

She was a Eucharistic minister for many years, delivering communion to nursing homes and homebound residents in her parish. She volunteered at the local food pantry several times a month and was part of the church's respite care group providing much-needed rest and downtime for the caregivers of Alzheimer's and dementia patients in the community.

It's ironic that my mother would become such a patient one day; it's even more ironic that I would become one of the caregivers so needing the rest she offered freely to others each month for years. She never would have wanted it that way. I know because she would often tell me about the families she had come to know, and she wondered aloud why so many families had to deal with this terrible illness and how they did it. She was happy to help them when she could even though she came home worn out from the experience and a little down and depressed after her respite activities.

Nonetheless, she made her activities fun by dressing up on various holidays such as Halloween and Christmas, and she danced with the members to music from long ago. I am comforted by the many pictures I found in her belongings highlighting her activities. She always had the attitude that there is always a way to make even the most difficult or mundane activity fun. She would often dress up like a clown and participate in her community's Fourth of July parade, Memorial Day parade, or umpteen activities I saw in the photos that unfortunately were never labeled with the event, date, or time. She always had a light, loving heart, and I am continually grateful for the many gifts she gave me over the years.

She never spoke about all the things she was involved in with the church or in the community. Many times over the years when she described her activities, I would think, *Didn't she just do that yesterday? Is she on another committee or headed to another luncheon, fashion show, or meeting? Mom, you should slow down.* Looking back now I believe these activities slowed her mental decline, and they provided her with grace and love from her many friends involved in the same activities.

Nana Nu held strong to tradition, and this provided guidance and direction for our family. In our family, religion and faith are one because she lived it. Advent, Lent, Easter, and Christmas were laden with wonderful memories and traditions that I treasure today. We all experienced baptism and First Holy Communion celebrations and fasting during Lent, and we attended Mass on Ash Wednesday, Holy Thursday, and Good Friday. We viewed the Stations of the Cross, prayed the Rosary, attended midnight mass on Christmas Eve, and sang traditional songs such as "Be Not Afraid", "On Eagle's Wings", and "Here I am Lord" (lyrics provided in the Appendix), which I still listen to frequently and find comfort in. I grew up with a rich fabric of religious tradition, and it has been a source of strength during good and bad times.

In addition to the religious traditions listed above and many others not mentioned, my mother incorporated many other traditions into our family life: special foods, a special Swedish drink known as Glogg (recipe provided in Appendix; I was always afraid she'd torch our house when making it), spritz cookies, Swedish textiles, and Swedish candles to name a few.

I learned of many of her activities, including various awards that she received, only after going through her things when she passed. She was honored as the volunteer of the month several times. That was Nana Nu. She was never boastful. It was the way she lived her life.

After she passed, as I was cleaning out Mom's desk, I found many magazine, newspaper, and Sunday church bulletin poems, words to songs she loved, quotes, and advice articles. It was as if I could hear

Mom's voice saying to me, "I left you these to find after I'm gone. I believe in what they say, and I hope you take the time to read them, Laura." Between the many unopened bank statements, unopened mail, and other old papers from years past, I found multiple references to angels in almost every place I looked—her desk, her jewelry box, her nightstand, and her closets and drawers.

The angel items were many, but each spoke to its existence and purpose and revealed stories about how angels have interceded in people's lives offering meaning and comfort. Her jewelry box was filled with angel pins and necklaces. I placed one very special angel pin on her dress during her wake right before she was buried. Her tombstone was inscribed with the words Angel on Earth, and anyone who knew her knew this to be true.

She was laid to rest holding a beautiful set of rosary beads that brought her much comfort over the years. Even during the last several months of her life while she was in the ALF, she received communion from the Eucharist ministers from the local Catholic Church. I am thankful for this, as I know it brought much comfort to her even in her final days. I know she felt bad about not attending church toward the end of her life because she would say, "I hope the good Lord understands that I didn't make it to church today. I'm just not feeling up to it." I confidently told her I thought it would be all right.

So what was Nana Nu's philosophy about religion and faith?

This is one area I did not have the opportunity to explore more deeply with my mother when I began asking her my soul-searching questions.

After much thought and reflection, however, I realized I didn't need to ask her because she lived it her entire life. I saw it in action. She modeled it for me every day. She taught me that life is not always easy, fair, clear, or understandable. Keep true to your beliefs even when the tide of public opinion or sentiment sways in a different direction or when people make fun of you or say things to hurt you. Keep your integrity and trust in the higher power—perhaps you will be the light that makes someone's day or their view of the world just a little better!

Life Questions, Life Lessons:

RELIGION

- What is the most important lesson you have learned about religion?
- Are religion and faith the same thing? If not, how are they different?
- What do you believe happens after you die?
- Do you believe in heaven?
- Do you believe in hell?
- Is prayer important?
- How do you pray?
- What traditions do you treasure regarding religion?
- What message or advice do you have about religion and faith?

Chapter Eight

HEALTH

*"A good laugh and a long sleep are
the best cures in the doctor's book."*
—Irish Proverb

W hen you don't have your health, you don't have much. If
you have health, you have wealth. I've come to believe this
completely! I know Nana Nu did.

My mother had her share of health issues over the years. She had a
cancer scare back in the 1980s and various other health concerns along
the way. She had a couple of falls, but we were lucky that nothing was
ever broken. By the time she passed away, she was taking multiple
medications, as is typical for most people her age. The average senior
is on thirteen different medications at any given time.

By the time my mother was in her eighties, I believe she had accepted her health as it was. My father religiously filled her pillboxes and tried to keep her on track taking them as her doctors prescribed. But if it was up to her, I believe she really didn't care about taking her pills. She had a live-and-let-live attitude.

Back in early 2008, my father and I made an urgent trip to the emergency room with Mom. Her breathing was labored. She was tired, lightheaded, and didn't want to get out of bed. She couldn't walk far without sitting down to rest. We knew she had heart issues, and this episode caused us great concern.

We arrived at the all-too-familiar emergency room, and Mom was ushered quickly to a bed in the ER for evaluation. It was very busy that day. The floor was buzzing with activity. One of the ER physicians whom we had grown to know and appreciate over the years came to her bedside. He wanted to run all types of tests, so off we went to various other areas of the hospital for evaluation.

After many hours and many tests, the doctor came to my mother's bedside to speak with us. Before he could launch into his evaluation, my mother looked him straight in the eye and said, "I know how to cure this problem, doctor."

The doctor looked down at the gray-haired lady in the bed and said, "Really? Tell me how."

She said, "Glogg."

The doctor repeated what she said. "Glogg—what is that?" He looked at Dad and me, and we just smiled. Mom proceeded to tell him it was a Swedish recipe made with several different forms of alcohol including port wine, whisky, and rum. She said that just a small glass of Glogg every day—heated up just a little bit—would cure most everything wrong with you. The doctor smiled, nodded his head, and said that they should teach that in medical school. Mom agreed.

She never was much of a drinker—except for a glass or two of Glogg each year at Christmas. Maybe Nana Nu was right. Perhaps we take life just a little too seriously, and we just need to slow down and have a drink.

Once we got Mom settled into her new apartment at the ALF, I took her for a new patient visit with a local physician who would be attending her going forward. He was a geriatrician, so he had a good deal of experience treating seniors. I knew Mom really didn't want to go, but it was important to become established with someone local. The doctor entered the room carrying an old-fashioned black doctor's bag.

The doctor asked all kinds of questions but mostly just let my mother talk. Talk she did. When she was done, the doctor said, "I think I have a pretty good idea of your mom's history." Yup, I bet he did. But he did ask her, "Do you exercise?"

My mom said, "Oh, yes, I ride my bicycle." I nearly fell off my chair again. Mom hadn't ridden a bicycle in nearly sixty years! I said so, and she said she used to ride a bicycle when she worked at the Piping Rock Country Club during the summer. *Yup, her long-term memory is what's working right now!* I thought.

It's certainly interesting the roads we take to navigate our health. Many choose traditional medicine, some choose more holistic approaches, and others choose nothing at all. Whichever way you go, our health certainly can play a very important part in how we interact with the world.

The questions on the next page will help you find out more about a person's view of health. The insights can be profound.

Life Questions, Life Lessons:

HEALTH

- What is the most important lesson you have learned about your health?
- What is the best way to maintain your health?
- Why are so many people sick?
- Do you believe that people take their health for granted?
- What advice do you have about health and wellness?

Chapter Nine

WEALTH AND MONEY

"They say it is better to be poor and happy than rich and miserable,
but how about a compromise like moderately rich and just moody?"
—Princess Diana of Wales (1961-1997)

*M*oney means different things to different people. Having it or not having it can change your perspective on life completely.

I know my mother, like most people, would often talk about winning the lottery. I don't recall her actually saying what she would do with the money once she received it, though. I think just having it in the bank would bring comfort to her, and that would be wealth in her eyes.

We never went on any big vacations. We rarely ate out at restaurants. We never drove new cars, for that matter. We always had used cars—some with very high mileage. But we always made it to where we needed to go. We never went hungry. We always had a wonderful Christmas with presents under the tree. I more often than not had hand-me-downs—bicycles, clothes, toys, and other stuff. It never bothered me. Back then, we were just like everyone else.

Mom used to say jokingly, "It's just as easy to love a rich man as it is to love a poor one!" I know she was trying to get a subtle, or not so subtle, message across, but I do believe that my mother defined wealth differently than most people do.

Having grown up during the Depression, I believe my mother had a healthy respect for money and what it means not to have it. She was very conservative in her spending habits and believed that you need to make wise choices so as not to be a burden financially on others. She made sure of that.

I remember visiting Mom over the years, and she always had the two local grocery stores' weekly fliers on the kitchen table next to her big black scissors that she would use to clip coupons. It wasn't uncommon for her to make a grocery list each week for each of her local grocery stores depending on who had the item she wanted on sale. I think there are few people, including me, who would ever go to this length to save money. Perhaps we should. I remember her talking about saving up green stamps at the grocery store to purchase various items that the store was selling. She was disciplined when it came to money; there was no doubt about that.

I believe my mother thought wealth had more to do with having just enough to live without worry. I know she played the lottery and forever told the story of how she made $25 on the first lottery ticket she ever bought, and in the years she purchased weekly tickets, she rarely won more than a few dollars. In the end, she certainly had enough to take care of herself, and she was well prepared for all her needs.

She donated generously to her church, her high school, the local police and firefighters' organizations, and to charities that help the victims of disasters around the world. I found many cancelled checks to support her incredible generosity throughout the years.

She even planned and saved for her journey home to heaven. She would often begin conversations with "After I'm gone..." and "It's important for you to know that when I die...." I always changed the subject. The thought of not having her in my life was too hard to imagine. She was a planner and a career bookkeeper. Her wishes for her final days and funeral were well documented by her in the prearranged funeral policy purchased years before.

She planned her wake and funeral down to the smallest detail including the songs that should be played in the church and the clothes she wanted to wear. Her blue dress—the dress she wore to my wedding nearly fifteen years earlier—was what she wanted to wear. She loved that dress, only wore it once, and if you knew Nana Nu, you know that blue was always her favorite color.

I remember vividly when my own grandmother lived with us when I was a child. My grandmother chose one of her dresses from her closet and told my mother to bury her in it when the time came. It was a dress she wore often, and there was nothing special about it. It was a polyester green and white knee-length dress. From that day forward, my grandmother never wore it again. I remember my mother saying to me that she would not choose that everyday dress—that her mother deserved a beautiful dress when she went to meet the Lord. When she died, my grandmother wore a beautiful dress. It wasn't green and white polyester.

My mother didn't want me to face the same issue. In addition to the instructions about what she was to wear, she left a handwritten letter telling me exactly where to find the prearranged funeral policy. She placed sticky notes around the house to remind me—in the medicine cabinets, in her purse, and on various papers on her desk. She even included a $250 allowance in the policy to cover the cost of the flowers she wanted. She didn't want to be a burden to anyone, and she certainly didn't want the policy she had purchased to go unused, as I had found documentation that she'd paid for it monthly over the course of several years.

Not only did she leave me with instructions for her funeral, but she also left me a handwritten letter on what her wishes were for the first twenty-four hours after she passed. Included in this letter was what I should do for my father in the event that she died first. I am happy to say I honored her wishes completely.

Having cared for both my grandmothers and a great aunt in their final days and being responsible for planning their funerals, my mother knew the toll that it takes both emotionally and financially. She planned it all from beginning to end—except, of course, for the fact that dementia would take her short-term memory away forever. In retrospect, however, perhaps she even planned for that since she left me multiple notes everywhere. Maybe she knew. I think she might have.

The next page highlights some questions you can ask to explore someone's views on wealth and money.

WEALTH AND MONEY

- What is the most important lesson you have learned about money?
- How do you define wealth?
- Are wealth and money the same thing?
- What advice do you have about money?
- Why does money cause so many hardships?
- What lessons did you learn about work?
- What advice do you have for finding a job or career you love?
- What is your message about work, wealth, and money?

Chapter Ten

HUMOR

"A person without a sense of humor is like a wagon without springs. It's jolted by every pebble on the road."
—**Henry Ward Beecher** (1813-1887), American clergyman

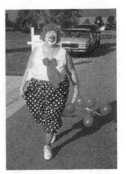

They say that laughter is the best medicine. I totally believe that, and Mom and I laughed often through the years! Even in her last months on earth, we had many funny times. I cherish them all.

Nana Nu would often ask, "What's wrong with me? Why can't I remember?" When she first started asking me these questions, I didn't want to tell her she had

Mom during a neighborhood parade. Circa 2002.

dementia or Alzheimer's disease. I thought it might upset her and make her angry or sad. So I would say that she was all right, or I would just change the subject. But she would ask again...and again...and again.

One day she asked, and finally I just said, "Mom, you've got Alzheimer's disease." I braced myself for her reaction. She said, "Oh..." and then she looked around the room and said, "Well, I'm eighty-two, you know. When you're eighty-two, it's okay to lose some of your memory!" We both laughed. From then on, whenever she would ask me why she couldn't remember things, I would just say, "You have Alzheimer's, but it's okay; you're eighty-two." She would love that and say, "You bet!"

> *Well, I'm 82 you know. When you're eighty-two, it's okay to lose some of your memory!*

On another occasion, I was in my car heading over to the ALF to see her, and my phone rang. I answered and it was Nana Nu wondering if I was coming over that night. I said yes and told her I had a surprise for her. She said "Really? I love surprises." I said yes and told her I was bringing her a frozen strawberry daiquiri. She was thrilled and said, "How fast can you get here?" I told her it would just be a few minutes, and she said "Hurry up!" and hung up.

An hour later, after just a few sips, she was sleeping like a baby. She loved it! The whole night was so much fun. Ironically, after she had passed and I was cleaning out her apartment, I found the green notebook I mentioned in chapter three. As I was thumbing through all the wonderful things we did together, I came to the entry dated Saturday, March 3 at 6:30 p.m., which I had written before I went home that night. It read:

*Today I came for a visit. We had strawberry daiquiris.
They were very good! We laughed a lot. Mom got new socks,
pants, and a shirt, too! Love you. See you tomorrow! Laura*

The best part of seeing that entry, and one that has forever touched my heart, was that just days before she died, unbeknownst to everyone, she wrote her own entry just below mine for that day. It read:

It's still March. Where is everybody? Sure could enjoy a daiquiri now!!

I look at that page often, and it helps me put life in perspective. I couldn't tell much else about that day, but I do know it was fun.

Another funny story happened just a month before she died. For Valentine's Day, I brought her flowers and a big helium balloon that said "Happy Valentine's Day!" During the weeks following February 14, the balloon lost much of the helium it originally contained and started to fall to the ground. One day while visiting her with my husband and children, I told her I wanted to clean up the vase and the balloon. She was fine with that, but instead of just forcing the last bit of helium out of the balloon and throwing it out, we decided to inhale the helium to see if we could make our voices change. Silly, I know, but what a great time we had doing it! My children, husband, and I all did it. Each person's voice changed so much. The best was when my husband, Tom, did it. His voice went from a bass to a soprano! We all laughed so much, and Mom laughed the most! We laughed such a deep belly laugh that we almost couldn't breathe. We had such a great time that my family still talks about it to this day.

There are so many other wonderful memories I have of Mom during the years. We really did have a wonderful time together, and they truly are some the best memories I have of her and us to this day!

When I think back on these wonderful memories, they still bring a sense of peacefulness and joy to my heart. In some strange way, our souls reconnect even though she is gone.

I encourage you to explore the issue of humor further with patients and your loved one. The next page has some questions that you might find helpful. Better yet, get creative and form your own funny memories to cherish and relive!

Life Questions, Life Lessons:

HUMOR

- What is the most important lesson you have learned about humor?
- What makes you laugh?
- Is humor important?
- Are there certain types of humor that are better than others?
- Are there times when humor is inappropriate? If so, when?
- What is your overall message about humor?

Part III

THE NEXT
CHAPTER

Chapter Eleven

THE BEGINNING

*M*ost books end with a conclusion. The last chapter of my book, however, is called "The Beginning" because that's what I believe it is. I believe that we are at the beginning of looking at Alzheimer's and dementia patients differently. We need to question the old approaches, redefine how to interact with these patients, and view them not as a burden, but as an incredible resource of life wisdom. I believe we need to change—not them.

In this book, I have provided some of my most treasured memories with my mother both good and not so good. Last month I celebrated my mother's first angelversary (my word for her anniversary) in heaven. In the past year, I have had many ups and downs as I have gone through the grieving process, but during this time I have been able to turn my own memories into life lessons. My goal for this chapter is to share them with you, and I hope you find them helpful on your journey.

- First and foremost, ask Alzheimer's and dementia patients a variety of open-ended, soul-searching questions and listen deeply to their responses.
- Be okay with silence and embrace its healing nature.
- Mom was right—growing old ain't for sissies.
- Pick your battles. Sometimes powdered coffee creamer is okay.
- No matter how much or how deeply you love someone, he or she has a finite time here on earth, just as we all do.
- Cherish your time together.
- Telling someone their loved one has died is one of the hardest things you might ever have to do.
- Don't ever turn your cell phone off completely in case someone is trying to reach you urgently. Put it on silent or vibrate mode instead.
- Prayer helps you get through the tough times.
- Sometimes people die alone. That might be how they wanted it—and the way it was supposed to be.
- Take deep breaths.
- When someone you love dies, it will change you forever.
- Take time to grieve—no matter how long that may be.
- Enjoy an evening walk, even if you need to go in a wheelchair, because it might be the last.
- Enjoy the sounds of birds and the beauty and sweet scents of flowers.
- Always hug and kiss your loved ones goodbye.
- The eyes truly are the windows of the soul. Look deeply into the eyes of the people who are important to you.
- Create a departing saying you quote every time you say goodbye. Let it become part of your legacy together.

- If possible, look into assisted living facility placement for your loved one or other forms of help such as in-home providers to alleviate caregiver burnout and stress.
- A change in living environment can really enhance the dynamic of your personal interactions.
- Hold hands.
- Don't let your caregiving situation reach the breaking point. Reassess the situation and make changes as needed.
- If you are not in a direct caregiving role, support those who are. You will never fully understand the burden that is placed on caregivers. Offer support and encouragement.
- If you are in a direct caregiving role, don't expect anyone who is not a caregiver to understand your burden. Seek out those who will listen and provide support.
- Think ahead for yourself regarding your long-term plans as you age. Plan, plan, plan and save, save, save!
- Laugh, sing, and talk.
- Remember that you can fly solo.
- Recognize anticipatory grief and reach out for help on your journey.
- The memories you are creating now will be the most vivid, at first, after your loved one passes. Older memories will come back over time and replace the most recent ones. Cherish them all.
- Access your loved one's wisdom and life lessons but realize that you too are creating your own in the process.
- Don't fall into the trap of believing everything you read and hear. No one has all the answers.
- Create your own approaches to dealing with your Alzheimer's/dementia patient.

- See the big picture.
- Don't waste time with small talk. Most of it doesn't matter.
- Recognize that time is ticking.
- Things always change.
- Your loved one has more wisdom than you know. Tap into it and cherish it!
- Continually look for new ways to interact with your loved one.
- You may also develop Alzheimer's and dementia. What would you like your caregivers to know? Write it down.
- Recognize that you encounter many people every day who are playing a caregiving role to someone with Alzheimer's, dementia, or another condition. A smile or kind word could really brighten his or her day!
- A new approach is often needed to confront a crisis or difficult situation.
- The nation is and will continue to struggle under the financial burden of Alzheimer's and dementia.
- Children may have a relative with Alzheimer's or dementia and not understand what is happening. Seek care and comfort for them, too.
- Don't assume it's easy to deal with aging parents when you have not yet been down that road with your own.
- Grandparents and parents are not the same.
- Plan and pay for your funeral. It is a significant burden to leave for someone else.
- Be supportive and respectful of caregivers. If they don't return your call right away, be understanding. Don't expect an update after every doctor appointment and at every turn in events. Reach out respectfully to caregivers, as there is often much on their minds.

- Send cards and flowers of encouragement to caregivers. It could mean the world to them on a difficult day!
- Purchase long-term care insurance and periodically upgrade your policy with the cost of living indexes if you are able.
- Don't assume any two patients are the same.
- Don't assume any patient is the same from minute to minute.
- Don't assume that just because you or another caregiver works in healthcare that you, he, or she always know what to do.
- Recognize denial.
- Having parents at two different functional levels is difficult. Find the best solution you can, but recognize that you may need to create a new approach to living that is best for both.
- When it's time to act, don't hesitate. Seize the moment and your energy. You will get through it. Run on adrenaline if you have to, but realize that it's not a good long-term approach.
- Have a spouse as a best friend and cherish his or her love.
- Talk to your children about the decline of their grandparents so they understand what is happening.
- Include your children in caring for your loved one, but don't overburden them with physical and emotional responsibility that they are unprepared to handle.
- Don't pack too much into your agenda on any given day.
- Alzheimer's and dementia patients will take on whatever mood or disposition they sense from you, so before walking into their room, put on a smile and show them love in your voice and in your actions.
- Try to leave your troubles at the door.

- Alzheimer's and dementia patients hate to take showers, so be creative to facilitate this task.
- Keep lots of cleaning supplies in the house.
- How you pitch something to someone can significantly alter his or her reaction to it.
- Research senior living options in your area. Keep in touch with them over time and get on their waiting list if they have one. This way you have a plan when and if the time is right for such a move.
- Put basic health and safety first for everyone's sake.
- Sometimes the parent and child roles are reversed. Sometimes they flip back and forth. Be flexible.
- Any problem can be changed, altered, or solved if you look at it from a new perspective.
- It may take several moves before you finally get your loved one in the right caregiving environment. Allow time for your loved one to settle in, but if he or she isn't happy, look for a new situation.
- Organize your important papers and make sure your caregivers and family know where they are.
- If you move your loved one, make sure to get copies of their medical records and keep a record for yourself.
- Choose a new primary care physician if you move and make sure to establish yourself as a new patient as soon as possible.
- Traditional wisdom doesn't have all the answers.
- Focus on your loved one and create the most meaningful lasting legacy possible. It will help them and you!
- Use your car as your own private sanctuary if you need to.
- Pray more.
- Lives can be touched even when you don't know much about another person.

- If someone is willing, able, and available to help you with caregiving, meet that person halfway. It helps not to drive the entire way when caregiving from a distance.

- Become a super sleuth in figuring out what is going on in an Alzheimer's and dementia patient's home.

- Seek help for daily caregiving tasks even if it's just sitting quietly to give you a break outside the home.

- Word search books can be fun and distracting if only for a short while. Have lots of them around so they are easily accessible.

- Getting back to basics can be a great goal—food, medication, and a safe, clean environment.

- Little white bathroom cups with stickers or sweet messages such as "Take me. I'm yours!" on them can entice someone to take her medications.

- Daily check-in calls may provide a sense of relief and comfort because you'll know everything is okay—even if only temporarily.

- Make sure to have the following documents and keep them updated: last will and testament, living wills, power of attorney, and healthcare proxy documents.

- Include patients and family members in conversations regarding legal matters and documents. This eliminates any suspicion that you are talking behind someone's back or keeping a patient or family member out of the decision-making process. You may be surprised that the Alzheimer's patient is able to comprehend the conversation on some level.

- Look for evidence that logical thinking and in-depth thought processes still exist. Sometimes these moments occur when you least expect it.

- Even after a patient answers one of your questions, remain silent, as they may add more to their response or explain their response in greater detail.
- Remember the equation: EXPERIENCES > MEMORIES > LIFE LESSONS > LIFE PURPOSE. See chapter four for additional information.
- Our culture is stuck on memories.
- We must focus on turning memories into life lessons.
- We must ask ourselves what we have learned from an experience.
- Time can be shorter than you realize.
- An assisted living facility environment can be a healing, open, and fresh environment for both the patient and the caregiver.
- Don't assume you know how the Alzheimer's and dementia patient will respond to various open-ended questions.
- A patient diary can be a wonderful tool to record memories of your time together.
- Maps can provide a tool to reliving memories of the past and facilitating the retrieval of life lessons.
- A dry erase board can be a fun and creative communication tool for drawing or writing short messages.
- When interacting with patients, everything is trial and error. The patient can change over time, so try different ideas from time to time.
- A phone in an ALF apartment can be a good way to stay connected, but patients may call you at odd times of day since their sleep cycles are often very different from the norm.
- Don't just be nice—be kind.
- Friendships are important.

- Patients often think their dreams are real and need you to help ground them.
- Life can be ironic in that you are drawn to activities that you may need in the future.
- Early religious beliefs and teachings are engrained in you forever.
- Even the most mundane and difficult task can be made fun with a little creativity.
- Family traditions are important for everyone. They become an important part of your life blueprint.
- Angels exist and guide us every day.
- Live your beliefs. They speak louder than words.
- Drink a little Glogg every once in a while (recipe in the Appendix). Don't forget to heat it up!
- Appreciate emergency room doctors and staff. They have a tough job.
- Don't take life too seriously. It's only temporary.
- Make wise money decisions.
- Wealth means different things to different people.
- Having money in the bank can bring comfort.
- Hand-me-downs are okay.
- Donate to worthy causes. Don't be boastful about it.
- When you're eighty-two, it's okay to lose your memory.
- Surprises are important even when you're eighty-two.
- Strawberry daiquiris are a good surprise.
- Little things can be the most fun.
- Laugh often.
- Be creative in your fun!
- If you are struggling with something that is not working, try to see it from a different perspective.

I will end this chapter—or should I say start "The Beginning"—with a beautiful Irish prayer:

An Irish Blessing

May the road rise up to meet you

May the wind be always at your back

May the sun shine warm upon your face

May the rains fall soft upon your fields

And until we meet again

May God hold you in the palm of his hand.

God's speed on your journey,

Laura

ACKNOWLEDGMENTS

Caring for my mother and then writing this book has been an astonishing journey filled with many emotions. From the deepest part of my soul, I want to thank:

- The Dear Lord for his infinite guidance and support, for without him, no journey would be possible or meaningful.
- My husband Thomas, whose patience and encouragement have been never-ending.
- My loving children, Benjamin and Christina, who seem to know precisely when I need a hug.
- My father for his trust in all the twists and turns on this journey.
- My ever-present angel, my mother Nana Nu, who proved to me that all things are possible and that the journey never ends!

A SPECIAL GIFT
ESPECIALLY FOR YOU!

For your *free* *Life Question Guide*
and other inspirational messages please visit:
www.LauraAnthonyAuthor.com

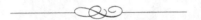

Tell a family member, friend and/or neighbor about this book!
It will make a world of difference in someone's life!

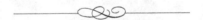

Share a little kindness today!

To receive your special gift, visit the website above.
You will then be prompted to enter your name & email address.
Once entered, click OK to receive your free gift!

Appendix

LIFE QUESTIONS

Chapter Five: Life

- What is the most important lesson you have learned in life?
- How would you define success?
- How would you define failure?
- What is happiness?
- How do you find happiness?
- What is your wish for humanity?
- How do you overcome difficulties in life?
- What is the best way to maintain balance in your life?
- What advice do you have for someone trying to find his or her path in life?
- What could the world use more of? Less of?
- What has always perplexed you about life?
- What is your ultimate message about life?

Chapter Six: Relationships

- What is the most important lesson you have learned about relationships?
- What makes a good marriage/partnership?

- What makes a happy family?
- What is the most important lesson to teach children?
- What surprises you most about people?
- How important are friends and family?
- How does someone be a good friend?
- What advice do you have for spouses, parents, and grandparents?
- Why do so many people struggle with relationships?
- What is the best way to deal with difficult relationships?
- What has always perplexed you about people?
- What is your overall message about relationships?

Chapter Seven: Religion and Faith

- What is the most important lesson you have learned about religion?
- Are religion and faith the same thing? If not, how are they different?
- What do you believe happens after you die?
- Do you believe in heaven?
- Do you believe in hell?
- Is prayer important?
- How do you pray?
- What traditions do you treasure regarding religion?
- What message or advice do you have about religion and faith?

Chapter Eight: Health

- What is the most important lesson you have learned about your health?
- What is the best way to maintain your health?
- Why are so many people sick?

- Do you believe that people take their health for granted?
- What advice do you have about health and wellness?

Chapter Nine: Wealth and Money

- What is the most important lesson you have learned about money?
- How do you define wealth?
- Are wealth and money the same thing?
- What advice do you have about money?
- Why does money cause so many hardships?
- What lessons did you learn about work?
- What advice do you have for finding a job or career you love?
- What is your message about work, wealth, and money?

Chapter Ten: Humor

- What is the most important lesson you have learned about humor?
- What makes you laugh?
- Is humor important?
- Are there certain types of humor that are better than others?
- Are there times when humor is inappropriate? If so, when?
- What is your overall message about humor?

On the following pages, I have included several items that have helped me along my journey. The three songs have brought me great comfort and healing because I know they were Nana Nu's favorite. I listen to them nearly every day. The "10 Commandments of Daily Living" poem was found in my mother's papers after she passed, and it is a testament to how she lived her life. Lastly, I've included Mom's recipe for Glogg. I know she would not only laugh at me for including this, but she would proclaim "Skal!" ("Cheers!" in Swedish) as she raised her glass high in the air and wished everyone health and happiness forever!

On Eagle's Wings

You who dwell in the shelter of the Lord,
Who abide in His shadow for life,
Say to the Lord, "My Refuge,
My Rock in Whom I trust."
And He will raise you up on eagle's wings,
Bear you on the breath of dawn,
Make you to shine like the sun,
And hold you in the palm of His Hand.
The snare of the fowler will never capture you,
And famine will bring you no fear;
Under His Wings your refuge,
His faithfulness your shield.
And He will raise you up on eagle's wings,
Bear you on the breath of dawn,

Make you to shine like the sun,
And hold you in the palm of His Hand.
You need not fear the terror of the night,
Nor the arrow that flies by day,
Though thousands fall about you,
Near you it shall not come.
And He will raise you up on eagle's wings,
Bear you on the breath of dawn,
Make you to shine like the sun,
And hold you in the palm of His Hand.
For to His angels He's given a command,
To guard you in all of your ways,
Upon their hands they will bear you up,
Lest you dash your foot against a stone.
And He will raise you up on eagle's wings,
Bear you on the breath of dawn,
Make you to shine like the sun,
And hold you in the palm of His Hand.
And hold you in the palm of His Hand.

Be Not Afraid

You shall cross the barren desert,
but you shall not die of thirst.
You shall wander far in safety,
though you do not know the way.
You shall speak your words in foreign lands,
and all will understand,
You shall see the face of God and live.
Be not afraid,
I go before you always,
Come follow me,

and I shall give you rest.
If you pass through raging waters
in the sea, you shall not drown.
If you walk amidst the burning flames,
You shall not be harmed.
If you stand before the pow'r of hell
and death is at your side,
know that I am with you, through it all
Be not afraid,
I go before you always,
Come follow Me,
and I shall give you rest.
Blessed are your poor,
for the Kingdom shall be theirs.
Blest are you that weep and mourn,
for one day you shall laugh.
And if wicked men insult and hate you, all because of Me,
Blessed, blessed are you!
Be not afraid,
I go before you always,
Come follow Me,
and I shall give you rest.

Here I Am, Lord

I, the Lord of sea and sky,
I have heard my people cry.
All who dwell in dark and sin
My hand will save.
I who made the stars of night,
I will make their darkness bright.
Who will bear my light to them?

Whom shall I send?
Here I am, Lord. Is it I, Lord?
I have heard You calling in the night.
I will go, Lord, if You lead me.
I will hold your people in my heart.
I, the Lord of snow and rain,
I have borne my people's pain.
I have wept for love of them.
They turn away.
I will break their hearts of stone,
Give them hearts for love alone.
I will speak my Word to them.
Whom shall I send?
I the Lord of wind and flame,
I will tend the poor and lame.
I will set a feast for them.
My hand will save.
Finest bread I will provide
'Til their hearts be satisfied.
I will give my life to them.
Whom shall I send?
Here I am, Lord. Is it I, Lord?
I have heard You calling in the night.
I will go, Lord, if You lead me.
I will hold your people in my heart.

The Ten Commandments for Daily Living
Blessed Pope John XXIII wrote these rules for himself

1. **Only for today,** I will seek to live the day positively without wishing to solve the problems of my life all at once.

2. **Only for today,** I will take the greatest care of my appearance; I will dress modestly; I will not raise my voice; I will be courteous in my behavior; I will not criticize anyone; I will not claim to improve or to discipline anyone except myself.

3. **Only for today,** I will be happy in the certainty that I was created to be happy, not only in the other world but also in this one.

4. **Only for today,** I will adapt to circumstances, without requiring all circumstances to be adapted to my own wishes.

5. **Only for today,** I will devote ten minutes of my time to do some good reading, remembering that just as food is necessary to the life of the body, so good reading is necessary to the life of the soul.

6. **Only for today,** I will do one good deed and not tell anyone about it.

7. **Only for today,** I will do at least one thing I do not like doing; and if my feelings are hurt, I will make sure that no one notices.

8. **Only for today,** I will make a daily plan for myself: I may not follow it to the letter, but I will make it. And I will be on guard against two evils: hastiness and indecision.

9. **Only for today,** I will firmly believe, despite appearances, that God cares for me as no one else who exists in this world.

10. **Only for today,** I will have no fears. In particular, I will not be afraid to enjoy what is beautiful and to believe in goodness.

Swedish Glogg: Nana Nu's Special Recipe

Ingredients

1 bottle (750 milliliters) Bordeaux Wine

1 bottle (750 milliliters) Port Wine

1 bottle (750 milliliters) Rye Whiskey

2 (8-inch) squares of cheesecloth

2 (6-inch) pieces of kitchen twine

2 cups white sugar cubes or "dots"

1 6oz. package mixed dried fruits

3 cinnamon sticks

1 tablespoon whole cloves

2 teaspoons cardamom

1 cup raisins

½ cup almonds- chopped

Directions

1. Make two cheesecloth bags by laying out the cheesecloth squares side by side. In the middle of one, place the mixed dried fruit, cinnamon sticks, cloves and cardamom. In the middle of the other, place the raisins and almonds. Gather the edges of the cheesecloth together and tie with kitchen twine to secure.

2. In a large stock pot with a lid bring 4 cups of water to a boil. Add the two cheesecloth bags and boil for 20 minutes. Allow to cool. Remove the spice bag and discard. Cut open the raisin and almond bag and put the contents into the water.

3. Add the Bordeaux wine, port wine and rye whiskey to the water and bring to a boil again.

4. Place the sugar cubes on a cookie cooling rack or metal grill and place across the top of the stock pot.

5. Carefully light the liquid in the pot with a long-handled match and let the flames melt the sugar into the stockpot. Be careful – the flames can shoot very high. When all the sugar has melted, remove the cookie cooling rack, put the lid on the stockpot to extinguish the flames, and turn off the heat. Let the mixture cool, covered, to room temperature, about 1 hour.

6. To store, pour cooled Glogg into large glass mason jars with lids (or the original bottles and cork). Keep upright in a cool dark place for up to one year.

7. To serve, pour Glogg into a saucepan and warm over low-medium heat until hot but not simmering, about 5 minutes. Ladle 3 ounces of warmed Glogg into a small coffee cup or small Swedish-style Glogg mug.

ABOUT THE AUTHOR

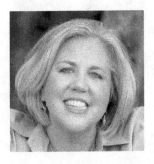 **Laura Anthony** is a healthcare professional with more than twenty-five years' experience in the hospital and home health arena. She received her bachelor's degree from SUNY Cortland in 1985 and her Master's of Public Health at the University of North Carolina at Chapel Hill in 1988. Since then, she has focused on improving the quality of life for patients and their families by working closely with hospitals, physicians, clinicians, and social workers.

Over the course of her career, Laura has had the opportunity to meet thousands of seniors. Her own real-life experience of caring for her mother, who had dementia, led her to question several preconceived notions about patients with Alzheimer's disease and dementia. She believes that *memories may fade, but deep, heartfelt* **life lessons** *still live on in a person with dementia and can be an incredible resource for us all.* Laura's goal is to help families and their communities unlock these lessons, enhance the quality of life with a loved one, and create a lasting legacy of hope and love.

Laura lives in Bradenton, Florida with her husband, Tom, and two children, Benjamin and Christina. To contact Laura, please visit her website at www.LauraAnthonyAuthor.com.

9 781614 487104